M

Dental An
and I

with Explanati
PG Entrance Examinations

MCQs on
Dental Anatomy, Histology and Embryology

with Explanations for BDS, MDS and PG Entrance Examinations

Satish Chandra
Director and Professor
Sardar Patel Postgraduate Institute of Dental and Medical Sciences, Lucknow

Ex-Professor and Head of the Postgraduate Department and Dean
Dental Faculty (Formerly KG Medical College and KG Medical University, UP
KG Dental University)
CSM Medical University, Lucknow

Ex-Professor, Dean, Head and Principal
DJ Postgraduate College of Dental Sciences and Research, Modinagar, UP
Ex-Professor, Dean, Head and Principal, Institute of Dental Sciences, Bareilly

Paper setter and Examiner for BDS, MDS and PGME Examinations in many
Universities
Ex-Member, Dental Council of India
Best Teacher Awardee

Shaleen Chandra
Professor and Head of the Department
Saraswati Postgraduate Dental College and Hospital, Lucknow
Ex-Professor and Head of the Department
Sardar Patel Postgraduate Institute of Dental and Medical Sciences, Lucknow
Ex-Assistant Professor, Rama Postgraduate Dental College and Hospital
and Research Centre, Kanpur
Ex-Lecturer, Dental Faculty (formerly KG Medical College, UP KG Dental
University and KG Medical University)
CSM Medical University, Lucknow
Ex-Lecturer, Budha Postgraduate Institute of Dental Sciences, Patna

Paper setter and Examiner of BDS, MDS and PGME Examinations in many
Universities

Girish Chandra
Rajendra Nagar Dental Clinic, Lucknow

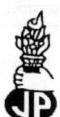

JAYPEE BROTHERS MEDICAL PUBLISHERS (P) LTD

New Delhi • Ahmedabad • Bengaluru • Chennai • Hyderabad
Kochi • Kolkata • Lucknow • Mumbai • Nagpur

Published by
Jitendar P Vij
Jaypee Brothers Medical Publishers (P) Ltd
B-3 EMCA House, 23/23B Ansari Road, Daryaganj, **New Delhi** 110 002, India
Phones: +91-11-23272143, +91-11-23272703, +91-11-23282021, +91-11-23245672
Rel: +91-11-32558559, Fax: +91-11-23276490, +91-11-23245683
e-mail: jaypee@jaypeebrothers.com,
Visit our website: www.jaypeebrothers.com

Branches

❑ 2/B, Akruti Society, Jodhpur Gam Road Satellite,
   Ahmedabad 380 015
   Phones: +91-79-26926233, Rel: +91-79-32988717, Fax: +91-79-26927094
   e-mail: ahmedad@jaypeebrothers.com
❑ 202 Batavia Chambers, 8 Kumara Krupa Road, Kumara Park East
   Bengaluru 560 001, **Phones:** +91-80-22285971, +91-80-22382956,
   080-22372664, Rel: +91-80-32714073, Fax: +91-80-22281761
   e-mail: bangalore@jaypeebrothers.com
❑ 282 IIIrd Floor, Khaleel Shirazi Estate, Fountain Plaza, Pantheon Road
   Chennai 600 008 , **Phones:** +91-44-28193265, +91-44-28194897
   Rel: +91-44-32972089, Fax: +91-44-28193231
   e-mail: chennai@jaypeebrothers.com
❑ 4-2-1067/1-3, 1st Floor, Balaji Building, Ramkote Cross Road,
   Hyderabad 500 095, **Phones:** +91-40-66610020, +91-40-24758498, Rel:+91-40-32940929,
   Fax:+91-40-24758499, e-mail: hyderabad@jaypeebrothers.com
❑ No. 41/3098, B & B1, Kuruvi Building, St. Vincent Road,
   Kochi 682 018, Kerala, **Phones:** +91-484-4036109, +91-484-2395739,
   +91-484-2395740, e-mail: kochi@jaypeebrothers.com
❑ 1-A Indian Mirror Street, Wellington Square
   Kolkata 700 013, **Phones:** +91-33-22651926, +91-33-22276404,
   +91-33-22276415, Rel: +91-33-32901926, Fax: +91-33-22656075
   e-mail: kolkata@jaypeebrothers.com
❑ Lekhraj Market III, B-2, Sector-4, Faizabad Road, Indira Nagar,
   Lucknow 226 016, **Phones:** +91-0522-3040553, +91-0522-3040554,
   e-mail: lucknow@jaypeebrothers.com
❑ 106 Amit Industrial Estate, 61 Dr SS Rao Road, Near MGM Hospital, Parel
   Mumbai 400 012, **Phones:** +91-22-24124863, +91-22-24104532
   Rel: +91-22-32926896, Fax: +91-22-24160828
   e-mail: mumbai@jaypeebrothers.com
❑ "KAMALPUSHPA" 38, Reshimbag, Opp. Mohota Science College, Umred Road
   Nagpur 440 009 (MS), **Phone:** Rel: +91-712-3245220
   Fax: +91-712-2704275, e-mail: nagpur@jaypeebrothers.com

MCQs on Dental Anatomy, Histology and Embryology

First Edition: **2007**

ISBN : **81-8448-176-4**

Typeset at   JPBMP typesetting unit
Printed at   Rajkamal Electric Press, B-35/9, G.T.Karnal Road, Delhi-33

Foreword

The progressive concept is changing very fast from subjective to objective. In many universities a part of the professional examination question papers contain objective type questions.

All the competitions contain only Multiple Choice Questions (MCQs). In MCQ type objective question papers, questions from the full course can be covered while only in subjective type question papers, it is not possible to cover the complete course of the subject, because out of an average of about 50 topics in a subject only 6 questions on 6 topics can be asked. When the question papers are of subjective type, students do only the superficial selective reading and lack the complete and deeper knowledge of the subject. With MCQ type of question papers the chances of leakage of the question papers are also very much reduced as they cover complete course of the subject and the students have to read complete course.

This book provides excellent and comprehensive coverage, covering all the aspects of the subject with unique and to the point explanations, which are in simple and easy language. This book is of great value to the students preparing for BDS and MDS and various competitive examinations.

Dr Anil Kohli
President
Dental Council of India

Preface

This book is written keeping professional and PG Dental entrance examinations in mind. Answers have been given with the explanations. It is based on the experience of many toppers regarding flying success in the examinations. This book will guide in preparations for examination. The questions in this book have been compiled after analyzing many question papers of previous years.

The secret of success in competitive examination lies in proper guidance and hard work. This book simplifies your preparation by making you work more efficiently. For the sake of convenience the MCQs have been divided subjectwise, one book on each major subject. Some allied subjects have been joined together.

All the books on MCQs will be true friends and a great asset for the candidates of dental professional examinations, the postgraduate dental entrance examinations and interview and also for practitioners.

The trend is very fast changing toward MCQs. These books will also be very useful for the students of graduate and postgraduate courses, as these contain questions, which are likely to be asked in periodical assessments during graduate and postgraduate courses and in final examinations.

For the preparation for examinations the aim of these books is to encourage the readers to detect areas of weakness in understanding the subject matter so that they may again study the textbooks for better and comprehensive review of the subject.

Every effort has been made to update all the books. All the books will be very useful for all the students and will prepare them to face any examination with full confidence.

Satish Chandra
Shaleen Chandra
Girish Chandra

Tips for Success

1. Start your preparations atleast one year in advance. Give six months for initial preparation (Reading Textbooks and solving MCQs), 4 months for final preparation (solving MCQs from books) and last two months for revision of MCQs.
2. Procure all study materials and finish subject by subject.
3. Plan your study hours.
4. Consult your seniors who have passed the examinations with a good score. Follow their advice but not blindly.
5. Read the textbook of the subjects thoroughly from the beginning to the end. Do not do selective reading except only in revision.
6. Be organised in your study
7. Aim for the top because you will invariably fall short.
8. Practice self-assessment tests and solve model test papers to know which chapters require revision and to get a feel of examination conditions.
9. Understand each chapter of each subject and attempt connected MCQs before proceeding to the next chapter. If you correctly answer less than 90% of MCQs, repeat the chapter.
10. Practise, practise and practise MCQs again and again with reasoning.
11. Time yourself while solving model test papers and examination question papers.
12. Relax and be tension-free while attempting questions in the examination.
13. Read the questions carefully to understand them, think and then answer.

Information and Suggestions

REMEMBER—You can do it. Always try for the top slots because if you aim for the sky, you would at least reach the hilltop.

You can do it and have to do it.

Tentative dates of various entrance exams		Approximate No. of seats available
All India PG	— Jan	130
AIIMS	— May/October	4
BHU	— July	2
PGI Chandigarh	— June/Nov	4
MAHE	— May	50
Various state/ College/ University entrances	— Jan to Dec	1000

The following is the approximate percentage of MCQs appeared in the various postgraduate entrance examinations in previous years.

Subject	No. of MCQs % age	Weeks required for revision Textbook	Weeks required for revision MCQ books
1. Purely preclinical	3	1	1
2. Applied preclinical	8	2	2
3. Oral and dental pathology and oral medicine	25	5	5
4. Oral and maxillofacial surgery	9	2	2
5. Periodontics	5	1	1
6. Prosthodontics and applied dental material	14	3	3
7. Conservative dentistry	8	2	2
8. Orthodontics	8	2	2
9. Dental radiology	3	2	2
10. Endodontics	5	2	2
11. Community dentistry	2	1	1
12. Gen. medicine and surgery	5	1	1
13. Pedodontics and preventive dentistry	5	1	1
Total	100	25	25

1. Only hard labour and vast knowledge are not enough but mastering the technique of taking MCQs examination is equally important.
2. First clear the basic fundamentals to have wider and better understanding of the subject. You must read the textbooks as much as possible.
3. Do not attempt the questions that you are not sure of. Negative marks due to guesswork always take you down in the merit list. Even 1 mark can change your merit tremendously.
4. It is better to leave a question rather than to attempt it wrongly.
5. Research in psychology has concluded that most of us mark the right choice first and due to second thoughts mark a wrong choice
6. The entrance examinations are to test the basic fundamental knowledge of the subject. Mostly the choices are straight forward and not to trick you. Answer each question from general principles rather than from exceptions.
7. Appear in all the entrance examinations in which you are eligible. You never know when luck may favour you.

Contents

MCQs on Dental and Oral Anatomy, Physiology and Occlusion

MCQs on Oral and Dental Histology and Embryology

MCQs on Dental and Oral Anatomy, Physiology and Occlusion

 Introduction

1. The rounded eminences prominent in the newly erupted incisors on the incisal edges are called:
   A. Tubercle
   B. Lobes
   C. Cusps
   D. Mamelons

2. The most important function of teeth is:
   A. To prepare food for swallowing and to facilitate digestion
   B. In speech and personal appearance
   C. Esthetics
   D. None of the above

3. The dentition which is involved in mastication of both vegetarian and nonvegetarian foods is known as:
   A. Omnivorous dentition
   B. Carnivorous dentition
   C. Herbivorous dentition
   D. Herbivorous and carnivorous dentition

4. The small elevation on some portion of the crown produced by an extra-formation of enamel is called as:
   A. Cusp
   B. Tubercle
   C. Cingulum
   D. Ridge

5. When a buccal and a lingual triangular ridge join, they form a:
   A. Transverse ridge
   B. Marginal ridge
   C. Incisal ridge
   D. None of the above

6. **The union of the triangular ridge of the distobuccal cusp and the distal ridge of the mesiolingual cusp of maxillary molar forms the:**
   A. Marginal ridge
   B. Oblique ridge
   C. Both of the above
   D. None of the above

7. **Three rounded protuberances found on the incisal ridge of newly erupted incisor teeth are called as:**
   A. Mamelons
   B. Cingulum
   C. Ridge
   D. None of the above

ANSWERS

1. **D.** Mamelon represents the lobe.

2. **A.** The teeth by the actions of cutting, shearing, milling and grinding prepare food for deglutition. The form of teeth is consistent with the function they have to perform.

3. **A.** The dentition of mammals is heterodont and diphyodont. The dentitions involved in mastication of animal and vegetable foods are known as carnivorous and herbivorous respectively.

4. **B.** Tubercle is a deviation observed from the normal form.

5. **A.** The transverse ridge crosses the occlusal surface of premolars and molars in a buccolingual direction.

6. **B.** Oblique ridge is found in permanent maxillary first molars and deciduous maxillary second molars.

7. **A.** Mamelons are the representative of lobes, which are the basic unit of tooth formation.

2 Dental Anthropology (Comparative Study of Dentition)

1. Which of the following stages is the simplest form of the tooth development?
   A. Reptilian stage (Haplodont)
   B. Early mammalian stage (Triconodont)
   C. Triangular stage (Tritubercular molar)
   D. Quadritubercular molar

2. The presence of continuously growing incisor is the prominent feature of the following:
   A. Carnivora
   B. Rodentia
   C. Artiodactyla
   D. Perissodactyla

3. Sexual dimorphism is seen in teeth of:
   A. Homo sapiens
   B. Great apes
   C. Homo erectus
   D. All of the above

ANSWERS

1. **A.** The dentition of reptiles is homodont and polyphyodont.

2. **B.**

3. **B.**

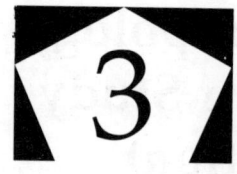

Development of Eruption of Teeth

3

1. **Which one of the following premolars does not develop from four lobes?**
   A. Maxillary first premolar
   B. Maxillary second premolar
   C. Mandibular first premolar
   D. Mandibular second premolar

2. **Maxillary incisors develop from which of following numbers of lobes?**
   A. 2
   B. 3
   C. 4
   D. 5

3. **A child normally at the age of 7 years has following number of teeth:**
   A. 16
   B. 20
   C. 24
   D. 28

4. **In the mandibular arch, canine erupts:**
   A. Before premolar
   B. After premolar
   C. Simultaneously with premolar
   D. None of the above

5. **The first evidence of calcification of permanent maxillary central incisor takes place at:**
   A. 3 to 4 months in intrauterine life
   B. 3 to 4 months after birth
   C. 1 year after birth
   D. 2 years after birth

6. **Eruption of permanent maxillary central incisor takes place at the age of:**
   A. 6-7 years
   B. 7-8 years
   C. 5-6 years
   D. 9-10 years

7. The mineralization of the crown of permanent maxillary central incisor is completed at the age of:
   A. 4-5 years
   B. 2-3 years
   C. 1-2 years
   D. 7-8 years

8. In permanent maxillary central incisor, root completion takes place after birth at the age of:
   A. 8 years
   B. 7 years
   C. 10 years
   D. 13 years

9. The first evidence of calcification of permanent maxillary lateral incisor appears at the age of:
   A. 8 months in intrauterine life
   B. 1 year after birth
   C. 2 years after birth
   D. 6 months after birth

10. Root completion takes place in permanent maxillary lateral incisor after birth at the age of:
    A. 11 years
    B. 9 years
    C. 7 years
    D. 6 years

11. Eruption of the permanent maxillary lateral incisor takes place after birth at the age of:
    A. 6-7 years
    B. 11-12 years
    C. 10-11 years
    D. 8-9 years

12. The first evidence of calcification of permanent mandibular central incisor appears at the age of:
    A. 3 to 4 months in intrauterine life
    B. 3 to 4 months after birth
    C. 5 to 6 months after birth
    D. 5 to 6 months in intrauterine life

13. The root completion of permanent mandibular central incisor takes place at the age of:
    A. 7 years
    B. 6 years
    C. 11 years
    D. 9 years

14. The crown completion of permanent mandibular central incisor takes place at the age of:
    A. 2 to 3 years
    B. 4 to 5 years
    C. 6 to 7 years
    D. 7 to 8 years

15. The eruption of permanent mandibular central incisor takes place at the age of:
    A. 6 to 7 years
    B. 4 to 5 years
    C. 7 to 8 years
    D. 8 to 9 years

16. The first evidence of calcification of permanent mandibular lateral incisor appears at the age of:
    A. 3 to 4 months of intrauterine life
    B. 6 to 8 months of intrauterine life
    C. 3 to 4 months after birth
    D. 3 to 4 years after birth

17. The root completion of permanent mandibular lateral incisor takes place at the age of:
    A. 8 years
    B. 7 years
    C. 6 years
    D. 10 years

18. Eruption of permanent maxillary canine takes place at the age of:
    A. 9 to 10 years
    B. 11 to 12 years
    C. 13 to 14 years
    D. 8 to 9 years

19. The root completion of permanent maxillary canine takes place at the age of:
    A. 9 to 10 years
    B. 11 to 12 years
    C. 13 to 15 years
    D. 10 to 11 years

20. In permanent maxillary canine, crown completion takes place at the age of:
    A. 6 to 7 years after birth
    B. 6 to 7 months in intrauterine life
    C. 8 to 9 months in intrauterine life
    D. 8 to 9 years after birth

21. Which tooth has same eruption time as that of the permanent maxillary canine ?
    A. Permanent mandibular second premolar
    B. Permanent mandibular first premolar
    C. Permanent maxillary first premolar
    D. Permanent maxillary second premolar

22. How many lobes are required for the development of maxillary premolars?
    A. 3 lobes
    B. 4 lobes
    C. 5 lobes
    D. 2 lobes

23. The first evidence of calcification of the maxillary first premolar takes place at the age of:
    A. 2 to 3 years after birth
    B. 3 to 4 years after birth
    C. 1½ to 1¾ years after birth
    D. At birth

24. Eruption of the maxillary first premolar takes place at the age of:
    A. 9 to 10 years
    B. 10 to 11 years
    C. 11 to 12 years
    D. 8 to 9 years

25. How many lobes are required for the development of mandibular second premolar?
    A. 4 lobes
    B. 5 lobes
    C. 3 lobes
    D. 6 lobes

26. How many lobes are required for the development of mandibular first premolar?
    A. 4 lobes   B. 5 lobes
    C. 3 lobes   D. 6 lobes

27. The mandibular second premolar develops from 5 lobes which are:
    A. 3 buccal and 2 lingual lobes
    B. 2 buccal and 3 lingual lobes
    C. 4 buccal and 1 lingual lobes
    D. 4 lingual and 1 buccal lobes

28. First evidence of calcification of permanent maxillary first molar is:
    A. 1 year   B. 2 years
    C. 6 years   D. At birth

29. In the maxillary arch the permanent canine generally erupts:
    A. Before the premolars
    B. After the premolars
    C. At same time as the premolar
    D. None of the above

30. At what age the calcification of deciduous teeth starts?
    A. Second month of fetal life
    B. Fourth month of fetal life
    C. Sixth month of fetal life
    D. Seventh month of fetal life

31. Which of the following permanent teeth appears in the maxillary arch before any deciduous teeth are lost?
    A. Lateral incisor
    B. Central incisor
    C. Second molar
    D. First molar

32. **At what age the complete deciduous dentition erupts in the oral cavity?**
    A. 2½ to 3 years
    B. 3 to 4 years
    C. 4 to 5 years
    D. 5½ to 6½ years

33. **Deciduous molars are replaced by which permanent teeth?**
    A. Permanent first molar
    B. Permanent second molar
    C. Premolars
    D. None of the above

34. **In permanent dentition which tooth erupts first in the oral cavity ?**
    A. Permanent first molar
    B. Permanent second molar
    C. Mandibular central incisor
    D. Maxillary central incisor

ANSWERS

1. **D.** Mandibular second premolar and first permanent molar develops from five lobes three buccal and two lingual.

2. **C.** The incisors develop from four lobes—three facial and one lingual. Most canines and premolars develop from four (or five) lobes—three facial lobes. Mandibular first premolar develops from four lobes. Mandibular second premolar develops from five lobes, three buccal and two lingual. The mandibular first molar develops from five lobes—three buccal and two lingual.

3. **C.** At (7 years ± 9 months) fourteen primary and ten permanent teeth will be present in mixed dentition.

4. **A.** Mandibular permanent canine erupts at 9 to 10 year of age and maxillary canine erupts at 11 to 12 years of age

5. **B.** Maxillary central incisor erupts at 7 to 8 years of age.

6. **B.** Refer to answer No. 5.

7. **A.**

Tooth	Age at which mineralization of crown is completed
Maxillary central incisor	– 4 to 5 years of age
Maxillary lateral incisor	– 4 to 5 years of age
Maxillary canine	– 6 to 7 years of age
Mandibular central incisor	– 4 to 5 years of age
Mandibular lateral incisor	– 4 to 5 years of age
Mandibular canine	– 6 to 7 years of age

8. **C.**

Tooth	Age of root completion
Maxillary central incisor	– 10 years
Maxillary lateral incisor	– 11 years
Maxillary canine	– 13 to 15 years
Mandibular central incisor	– 9 years
Mandibular lateral incisor	– 10 years
Mandibular canine	– 12 to 14 years

9. B. *Tooth*   *Age at first evidence of calcification*

Maxillary central incisor   – 3 to 4 months

Maxillary lateral incisor   – 1 years of age
Maxillary canine   – 4 to 5 months
Mandibular central incisor   – 3 to 4 months
Mandibular lateral incisor   – 3 to 4 months
Mandibular canine   – 4 to 5 months

10. A. Refer to answer No. 8

11. D. *Tooth (Permanent)*   *Eruption age*
Maxillary central incisor   – 7 to 8 years
Maxillary lateral incisor   – 8 to 9 years
Maxillary canine   – 11 to 12 years
Mandibular central incisor   – 6 to 7 years
Mandibular lateral incisor   – 7 to 8 years
Mandibular canine   – 9 to 10 years

12. B. Refer to answer No. 9

13. D. Refer to answer No. 8

14. B. Refer to answer No. 7

15. A. Refer to answer No. 11

16. C. Refer to answer No. 9

17. D. Refer to answer No. 8

18. B. Refer to answer No. 11

19. C. Refer to answer No. 8

20. A. Refer to answer No. 7

21. A. *Tooth*   *Eruption*
Maxillary first premolar   – 10 to 11 years
Maxillary second premolar   – 10 to 12 years
Mandibular first premolar   – 10 to 12 years
Mandibular second   – 11 to 12 years
premolar

Also refer to answer No. 11.

22. B.

Tooth (Permanent)		No. of lobes	
		Facial	Lingual
Incisor	–	3	1
Canines	–	3	1
Maxillary premolars	–	3	1
Mandibular first premolar	–	3	1
Mandibular second premolar	–	3	2
Mandibular first molar	–	3	2

23. C.

Permanent tooth		Age at first evidence of calcification
Maxillary first premolar	–	1½ to 2 years of age
Maxillary second premolar	–	2 to 2½ years of age
Maxillary first molar	–	At birth
Mandibular first premolar	–	1½ to 2 years of age
Mandibular second premolar	–	2¼ to 2½ years of age
Mandibular first molar	–	At birth

24. B.

Permanent tooth	Eruption age
Maxillary first premolar	– 10 to 11 years
Maxillary second premolar	– 10 to 12 years
Maxillary second molar	– 12 to 13 years
Mandibular first premolar	– 10 to 12 years
Mandibular second premolar	– 11 to 12 years
Mandibular second molar	– 11 to 13 years

25. B. Refer to answer No. 22

26. A. Refer to answer No. 22

27. A. Refer to answer No. 22

28. D. Refer to answer No. 23

29. B. Permanent maxillary canine erupts of the age of 11 to 12 years while maxillary first and second premolars erupt at the age of 10 to 11 years and 10 to 12 years respectively.

30. **B.** *Primary tooth*   *First evidence of calci-*
fication (weeks in utero)

- Maxillary
  Central incisor – 14 (12 to 16)
  Lateral incisor – 16 (15 to 16.5)
  Canine – 17 (15 to 18)
  First molar – 15.5 (14.5 to 17)
  Second molar – 19 (16 to 23.5)
- Mandibualr
  Central incisor – 14 (13 to 16)
  Lateral incisor – 16 (15 to 17)
  Canine – 17 (16 to 18)
  First molar – 15.5 (14.5 to 17)
  Second molar – 18 (17 to 19.5)

31. **D.** Permanent mandibular first molars are the first teeth to emerge through the gingiva at approximately 6 years of age and the second permanent tooth to emerge into the oral cavity is the mandibular central incisor at 6 to 7 years of age, which is first succedaneous tooth to emerge through the gingiva.

32. **A.** The deciduous second mandibular molar erupts at a mean age of 27 months and the deciduous second maxillary molar erupts at a mean age of 29 months (range 24 to 33 months) of age.

33. **C.** Premolars are succedaneous teeth and are present only in permanent dentition in place of deciduous molars.

34. **A.** The first teeth of permanent dentition to emerge through the gingiva are the first molars. Because eruption occurs at approximately 6 years of age, the teeth are called "6-year molars."

4   Tooth and Surface Identification

1. How many line angles are there in the crowns of mandibular first molar?
   A. 4 line angles
   B. 6 line angles
   C. 8 line angles
   D. 10 line angles

2. How many point angles are there in the anterior teeth?
   A. 3
   B. 4
   C. 5
   D. 6

3. Tooth number 29 in universal numbering system indicates:
   A. Upper right first premolar
   B. Upper right second premolar
   C. Lower right second premolar
   D. Lower right first premolar

4. Tooth number 34 indicates left lower first premolar in which of the following system of notations:
   A. Universal numbering system
   B. FDI system
   C. International System of Tooth Notation
   D. Both (B) and (C)

ANSWERS

1. C. Line angles in posterior teeth are eight in number.

2. B. A point angle is formed by the junction of three surfaces or three line angles. Posterior and anterior teeth have four point angles.

3. C. For permanent teeth in universal numbering system number 1 to 32 are used. It starts with 1 for maxillary right third molar going around the arch to the upper left third molar as 16. Left mandibular third molar becomes 17, around the lower arch the number increases to 32, which is lower right third molar.

4. B. In two digit or FDI or the International System of Tooth Notation, each quadrant is represented by number as following:

Upper right 1	2	Upper left
Lower right 4	3	Lower left

Therefore, the numbering of permanent dentition according to FDI system is as follows:

Upper right	Upper left
18 17 16 15 14 13 12 11	21 22 23 24 25 26 27 28
48 47 46 45 44 43 42 41	31 32 33 34 35 36 37 38
Lower right	Lower left

 **Deciduous (Primary) Teeth**

1. **In the deciduous teeth center of formation of each lobe is located:**
   A. At the center of the cusp
   B. At the cusp tip
   C. At the base of the cusp
   D. In the developmental groove separating the cusps

2. **Which of the following teeth is/are called succedaneous?**
   A. Permanent incisor and canine
   B. Premolars
   C. Premolars and permanent canine
   D. All of the above

3. **The pulp chambers are relatively larger in proportion of the crowns in the:**
   A. Deciduous teeth
   B. Young permanent teeth
   C. Old aged permanent teeth
   D. Both (A) and (B)

4. **The teeth in which roots are relatively longer, more slender and more flared are?**
   A. Permanent molars
   B. Premolars
   C. Deciduous molars
   D. All of the above

5. **The deciduous mandibular second molar has resemblance with which of the following tooth?**
   A. Maxillary first premolar
   B. Permanent maxillary first molar
   C. Permanent mandibular first molar
   D. Permanent maxillary second molar

6. How many supplemental cusp is/are found on the deciduous maxillary second molar?
   A. 2
   B. 3
   C. 1
   D. 4

7. Oblique ridge is predominantly observed on the:
   A. Deciduous maxillary second molar and permanent maxillary first molar
   B. Maxillary first molar and second molar
   C. Mandibular first molar only
   D. Deciduous mandibular first molar and permanent mandibular first molar

8. Oblique maxillary ridge which is found on the maxillary first molar and deciduous second molar joins which cusps:
   A. Mesiolingual cusp with the distobuccal cusp
   B. Mesiobuccal cusp with the distobuccal cusp
   C. Mesiobuccal cusp with the distolingual cusp
   D. None of the above

9. The deciduous mandibular second molar has characteristics that resemble which of the following tooth:
   A. Permanent mandibular first molar
   B. Deciduous maxillary first molar
   C. Permanent mandibular second molar
   D. Deciduous mandibular first molar

10. The deciduous dentition remains intact until a child is about the age of:
    A. 3 years
    B. 4 years
    C. 5 years
    D. 6 years

11. How many well-developed cusps are found on the deciduous maxillary second molar?
    A. 3
    B. 2
    C. 4
    D. 5

ANSWERS

1. **B.**   Center of formation of tooth is called a lobe.

2. **D.**   The teeth, which develop and erupt in the place of respective deciduous teeth, are called succedaneous teeth.

3. **D.**   The size of the pulp cavity depends on the age of the tooth and its history of trauma. Secondary dentine is formed continuously throughout the life of the tooth as a normal process, as long as the vitality of the tooth is maintained. Therefore, the size of the pulp cavity is much larger in young individual than in an adult.

   Because of the thinner dentine and enamel in deciduous teeth, the pulp cavities are much larger in proportion to the overall size of teeth.

4. **C.**   The roots of deciduous anterior teeth are narrower mesiodistally and proportionally longer as compared to crown size than the roots of the permanent anterior teeth.

5. **C.**   Deciduous mandibular second molar is smaller in size than permanent mandibular first molar and also has a more prominent mesial cervical ridge, the roots are more slender and more widely spread.

6. **C.**   Deciduous maxillary second molar has one supplemental cusp called cusp of carabelli.

7. **A.**   Deciduous maxillary second molars are similar in most respects, with the cusp, ridges and fossa corresponding to those of permanent first molars.

8. **A.**   Distal to the oblique ridge is the distal fossa, which contains the distal developmental groove. This groove acts as a line of demarcation between the mesiolingual and distolingual cusps and continues on to the lingual surface as the lingual developmental groove.

9. **A.**   Refer to answer No. 5

10. D. The primary dentition is complete at about 2½ years of age, and no obvious intraoral changes occur until the eruption of the first permanent molar, commonly called the 6 year molar, makes its appearance in the month before any if the primary teeth are lost.

11. C. Deciduous maxillary second molar resembles permanent maxillary first molar tooth.

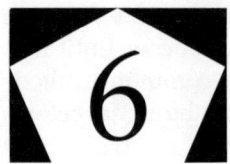

Physiology of Dentition

1. The center of the sphere in the curve of Monson, lies at:
   A. Nasion
   B. Bregma
   C. Glabella
   D. Lambda

2. The relative position of contact area in the facial view of teeth is demonstrated:
   A. Cervicoocclusally
   B. Buccolingually
   C. Both of the above
   D. None of the above

3. In teeth the curvature of cervical line is:
   A. More mesially than distally
   B. More distally than mesially
   C. Same mesially and distally
   D. Varies both mesially and distally

4. In an occlusal view of the teeth, contact point in posterior teeth is:
   A. Centered buccolingually
   B. Located buccally to the center
   C. Located lingually to the center
   D. Has no relation

5. When all the teeth are viewed facially the schematic outlines of crown are:
   A. Trapezoidal, with the longest uneven side being the incisal or occlusal surface
   B. Trapezoidal, with the longest uneven side being the cervical region
   C. Trapezoidal, with the shortest uneven side being the occlusal surface
   D. Rhomboidal in outline

6. Which of the following teeth surfaces appear rhomboidal in outline ?
   A. Proximal surfaces of maxillary posterior teeth
   B. Proximal surfaces of mandibular posterior teeth
   C. Facial surfaces of all teeth
   D. Proximal surfaces of anterior teeth

7. When anterior teeth are viewed from the proximal aspect they appear?
   A. Rhomboidal
   B. Trapezoidal
   C. Triangular
   D. None of the above

8. The compensating curvature of maxillary arch is:
   A. Convex
   B. Concave
   C. Flat plane
   D. None of the above

9. The interproximal space between the teeth is filled with the gingival tissues. The tissues is/are called as:

   A. Interdental papilla
   B. Intradental space
   C. Gingival papilla
   D. Both (A) and (C)

10. Which of the following is correct about curvature of the mandibular teeth?
    A. It is always concave
    B. Sometimes it is convex or concave
    C. It is always convex
    D. No correct knowledge about curvature

ANSWERS

1. **C.** Monson in 1920 proposed that on an average in adults the shape of the mandibular arch conforms itself to a part of sphere of 10.16 cm (4 inches) radius with its center at the glabella.

2. **A.** The incisal or occlusal views will demonstrate the faciolingual relative positions of the contact areas.

3. **A.** The curvature of the cervical line in most teeth is about 1 mm more mesially than distally.

4. **B.** Generally, anterior teeth have their contact areas centered labiolingually.

5. **A.** The shortest of the uneven side represent the bases of the crowns of the cervices.

6. **B.** The rhomboidal outline inclines the crowns lingual to the root bases, bringing the cusps into proper occlusion with the cusps of their maxillary opponents.

7. **C.** The base of the triangle is represented by the cervical portion of the crown, and the apex by the incisal ridge.

8. **A.** Curve of Wilson for the mandibular teeth is concave and that for the maxillary teeth is convex.

9. **D.** The interproximal spaces are triangular. Spaces between the anterior teeth, which are formed by proximal surfaces facing each other.

10. **A.** When seen from the anterior aspect with the mouth slightly open, the cusp tips of posterior teeth follow a gradual curve from the left side to the right side. The curve of the maxillary arch is convex and that of the mandibular arch is concave. This curve is known as curve of Wilson.

Physiologic Form of Teeth in Relation to Functions and Periodontium

1. **In teeth embrasures are:**
   A. Wider lingually than facially
   B. Wider facially than lingually
   C. Same facially and lingually
   D. None of the above

2. **In mandibular teeth all contact areas are centered buccolingually** *except:*
   A. Distal contact on second premolar
   B. Mesial contact on first molar
   C. Distal contact on first molar
   D. Distal contact on canine

3. **In permanent mandibular posterior teeth the maximum curvature is found at:**
   A. Cervical third of lingual surface
   B. Middle third of lingual surface
   C. Cervical third of buccal surface
   D. Middle third of buccal surface

4. **In maxillary permanent teeth the cervical curvature observed are:**
   A. More buccally than lingually
   B. More lingually than buccally
   C. Same buccally and lingually
   D. None of the above

5. **At the age of eight years in permanent central incisor the gingival line:**
   A. Follows the curvature of the cervical line
   B. Is same as cervical line
   C. Is located at the same height as the cervical line
   D. None of the above

6. The lingual inclination of the mandibular molars forms the basis of:
   A. Curve of Spee
   B. Curve of Wilson
   C. Curve of Monson
   D. None of the above

7. The occlusal view demonstrates the relative position of contact area:
   A. Faciolingually
   B. Cervico-occlusally
   C. Has no relation with contact area
   D. None of the above

8. The contact area between maxillary central incisors is located at:
   A. Incisal third
   B. Junction of incisal and middle third
   C. Middle third
   D. Middle of middle third

9. The contact area in the entire mandibular anterior region cervico-occlusally is at:
   A. Incisal third
   B. Junction of incisal and middle third
   C. Middle of middle third
   D. Cervical third

10. The only tooth wider lingually than buccally is:
    A. Maxillary second premolar
    B. Maxillary first molar
    C. Mandibular first molar
    D. Maxillary second molar

11. The only tooth other than maxillary third molar which has only one antagonist is:
    A. Mandibular central incisor
    B. Mandibular lateral incisor
    C. Mandibular second premolar
    D. Mandibular third molar

12. **The largest embrasure in the dental arch is:**
    A. Between maxillary canine and first premolar
    B. Between maxillary lateral incisor and canine
    C. Between maxillary central and lateral incisor
    D. Between mandibular canine and first premolar

13. **The curvatures present in tooth crowns are:**
    A. At the cervical thirds facially and middle thirds lingually
    B. At the cervical thirds facially and cervical thirds lingually
    C. At the middle thirds facially and cervical thirds lingually
    D. At the middle thirds facially and middle thirds lingually

14. **In the labial view contact areas of anterior teeth are in the incisal third of the crown. An *exception* to this rule is the:**
    A. Mesial contact area of maxillary canine
    B. Distal contact area of maxillary canine
    C. Mesial contact area of mandibular lateral incisor
    D. Distal contact area of mandibular lateral incisor

15. **The alveolar crest and interdental septum can be altered by:**
    A. Tilting of tooth
    B. Drifting of tooth
    C. Changing the height of the gingivoenamel junction
    D. All of the above

16. **Cervical line contours are closely related to the attachment of gingiva at the neck of the tooth. The greatest contours of cervical lines and gingival attachments occur on:**
    A. Distal surface of anterior teeth
    B. Distal surface of posterior teeth
    C. Mesial surface of anterior teeth
    D. Mesial surface of posterior teeth

17. **In the formation of interdental space:**
    A. Apex of triangle is formed by contact area
    B. Base of triangle is formed by contact area
    C. Apex of triangle is formed by alveolar bone
    D. None of the above

18. **The height of attachment is dependent on:**
    A. Curvature of cervical line
    B. Height of contact area
    C. Height of alveolar bone
    D. All of the above

19. The average normal separation between enamel and alveolar bone at the age of twenty years is:
    A. 0.5 to 1 mm
    B. 1 to 1.5 mm
    C. 0.5 to 1.5 mm
    D. 1.5 to 2 mm

20. Normally interproximal spaces between the teeth are triangular shaped spaces filled by gingival tissue. The base of the triangle is towards the:
    A. Alveolar process
    B. Proximal surfaces of contacting teeth
    C. Area of contact
    D. None of the above

21. The function of embrasure is/are mainly:
    A. To make spillway for the escape of food during mastication
    B. To prevent food from being forced through the contact area
    C. All of the above
    D. None of the above

22. In maxillary teeth, contact areas are present mesially on both central incisors in the:
    A. Incisal third of the crown
    B. Middle third of the crown
    C. At the junction of incisal and middle thirds of the crown
    D. Cervical third of the crown

23. In maxillary teeth, the distal contact area on lateral incisor is approximately present at the:
    A. Incisal third of the crown
    B. Middle third of the crown
    C. At the junction of incisal and middle third of the crown
    D. At the junction of cervical and middle third of the crown

24. In maxillary teeth, the mesial contact area on the canine is present at the:
    A. Junction of incisal and middle third
    B. Junction of middle and cervical third
    C. At the middle third of the crown
    D. None of the above

25. **In maxillary teeth, the contact area present between the first and second premolars is present at:**
    A. Occlusal third of the crown
    B. Middle third of the crown
    C. At the junction of the middle and cervical third of crown
    D. At the junction of the occlusal and middle third of crown

26. **In maxillary teeth, the contact areas present between first and second molars and between the second and third molars are present at the:**
    A. Same position
    B. Different position
    C. All of the above
    D. None of the above

27. **What is the position of the mesial contact area between the mandibular central incisors?**
    A. At the incisal third of the crown
    B. At the middle third of the crown
    C. At the junction of incisal and middle thirds of the crown
    D. None of the above

ANSWERS

1. **A.** Because the most of the posterior teeth have contact areas slightly buccal to the center bucco-lingually and all crowns except maxillary first molar, converge lingually more than facially from contact areas.

2. **B.** The mesial contact area of the first molar is located farther buccally than any of the other contact areas on mandibular posterior teeth.

3. **B.** Mandibular first molar has a curvature of approximately 1mm lingually, with the crest of curvature at the middle third.

4. **C.** Normal curvature from the cementoenamet junction to the crest of contour is approximately 0.5 mm in extent and it is fairly constant for maxillary teeth, labially or buccally and lingually

5. **A.** Cemento enamel junction and epithelial attachment tend to follow the same curvature even though the epithelial attachment may be higher on the crown on its enamel surface.

6. **B.** Curvature of the mandibular teeth is concave and that of the maxillary teeth convex.

7. **A.** Refer to answer No. 3

8. **A.** Since the mesioincisal third of maxillary central incisor approaches a right angle, the incisal embrasure is very slight.

9. **A.** The mesioincisal angle of the canine is more rounded than the other mandibular anterior teeth.

10. **B.** Mesiolingual and distolingual embrasures of maxillary first molar are almost similar in size, even though the tooth makes contacts with two teeth that are dissimilar lingually.

11. **A.** Mandibular central incisor is the smallest tooth of the dentition.

12. **A.**   The canine and first premolar contact is the transitional zone between anterior and posterior segments of teeth.

13. **A.**   These contours can deflect food material away from the gingival margins during mastication.

14. **B.**   The maxillary canine has a long distal slope to its cusp, which puts the distal crest of curvature of the center of the middle third of the crown. The contact area is, therefore, at the middle third of crown.

15. **D.**   Bone is biologically a highly plastic tissue. It is this biologic plasticity that enables the orthodontist to move teeth without disrupting their relations to the alveolar bone.

16. **C.**   The six anterior teeth, both maxillary and mandibular, when compared with posteriors, exhibit the greatest curvature.

17. **A.**   The base of the triangle is formed by the alveolar process.

18. **B.**   The height of normal gingival tissue, mesially and distally on approximating teeth is directly dependent upon the heights of the epithelial attachment on these teeth.

19. **B.**   The distance from the cementoenamel junction to the crest of the alveolar bone as seen radiographically is 1 to 1.5 mm in a normal occlusion in the absence of disease.

20. **A.**   Apex of the triangle is formed by area of the contact.

21. **C.**   When teeth wear down to the contact area so that no embrasure remains, especially in the incisors, food is pushed into the contact area even teeth are not mobile.

22. **A.**   Normally, contact points are never located more cervically than in the middle of the tooth crowns.

23. **C.**   The form of maxillary lateral incisor and canine creates an embrasure that is more open than the embrasure between central and lateral incisors.

24. A. The canines are shaped so that they act as a catalyst between anterior and posterior teeth.

25. D. The contact of maxillary first and second premolars is nearly level with that of the canine and the first premolar.

26. A. Because the molars become progressively shorter from the first to the third, the centers of the contact areas drop cervically also.

27. A. The incisal embrasure between maxillary central incisors is very slight.

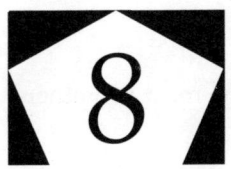 **Permanent Maxillary Incisors**

1. Which of the following anterior teeth is widest mesiodistally?
   A. Mandibular central incisor
   B. Mandibular canine
   C. Maxillary canine
   D. Maxillary central incisor

2. Which of the permanent tooth has greatest variation in form (except third molar)?
   A. Permanent mandibular premolar
   B. Permanent maxillary central incisor
   C. Permanent maxillary lateral incisor
   D. Permanent mandibular lateral incisor

3. The labial surface of maxillary central incisor than the maxillary lateral incisor and canine is:
   A. More convex
   B. Less convex
   C. Flat
   D. None of the above

4. The incisal edges are usually labial to the root axis line in:
   A. Mandibular incisors
   B. Maxillary incisors
   C. Both A and B
   D. None of the above

5. The only maxillary tooth whose root is equally thick at the cervix in both the directions mesiodistally and faciolingually is :
   A. Maxillary central incisor
   B. Maxillary lateral incisor
   C. Maxillary canines
   D. Maxillary first premolars

ANSWERS

1. **D.** The maxillary central incisors are the most prominent teeth in the mouth.

2. **C.** If the variation is too great, it is considered a developmental anomaly such on peg laterals. One type of malformed maxillary lateral incisor will have a large pointed tubercle as part of the cingulum, some will have deep developmental groves, which extend down on the root lingually with a deep fold in the cingulum; and some with show twisted roots, distorted crowns and so forth.

3. **B.** The crown of maxillary central incisor is symmetrical and regular having an almost straight edge. The distal side is very slightly curved. The mesioincisal angle is acute and the distoincisal angle is obtuse.

4. **B.** Maxillary incisors can be distinguished from mandibular incisors by arch characteristics.

5. **B.** The dimension is 6 to 6.4 mm. The roots of seven other maxillary teeth are thicker faciolingually than mesiodistally.

9 Permanent Mandibular Incisors

1. Which permanent tooth has smallest mesiodistal dimension?
   A. Maxillary lateral incisor
   B. Mandibular central incisor
   C. Mandibular lateral incisor
   D. Maxillary central incisor

2. Which of the following permanent teeth is smallest in volume in the dental arch?
   A. Mandibular central incisor
   B. Mandibular lateral incisor
   C. Maxillary lateral incisor
   D. Mandibular second premolar

3. The most symmetrical tooth in the dentition is:
   A. Maxillary central incisor
   B. Mandibular canine
   C. Mandibular central incisor
   D. Maxillary canine

4. The crown of which tooth is slightly tilted distally on the root axis and tapers lingually slightly in the middle and moderately in the cervical thirds?
   A. Mandibular central incisor
   B. Mandibular lateral incisor
   C. Maxillary central incisor
   D. Maxillary lateral incisor

ANSWERS

1. **B.**   The mesiodistal diameter of mandibular central incisor is about 5 mm and that of mandibular lateral incisor is about 5.5 mm.

2. **A.**   Normally, the mandibular central incisor is the smallest tooth in the dental arches.

3. **C.**   The only difference is the greater mesial than distal curvature of the cervical line. The mesial and distal outlines of the crown are almost straight.

4. **B.**   The mesial marginal ridge of mandibular lateral incisors is slightly longer than distal marginal ridge.

Permanent Canines

1. Which of the following permanent teeth is the longest tooth in the dental arch?
   A. Maxillary first molar
   B. Mandibular first molar
   C. Maxillary central incisor
   D. Maxillary canine

2. The root of which of the following permanent teeth is the longest?
   A. Palatal root of the permanent maxillary first molar
   B. Mesial root of the permanent mandibular first molar
   C. Buccal root of the permanent maxillary first premolar
   D. Root of the permanent maxillary canine

3. The mesiodistal width of crown of permanent mandibular canine is:
   A. 6 mm
   B. 7 mm
   C. 8 mm
   D. 8.5 mm

4. Which permanent tooth is the 'cornerstone' of dental arch?
   A. Maxillary second molar
   B. Mandibular first molar
   C. Maxillary canine
   D. Mandibular canine

5. Which tooth has the largest crown length?
   A. Permanent mandibular canine
   B. Permanent maxillary first premolar
   C. Mandibular second premolar
   D. Permanent maxillary central incisor

6. **Major portion of canine fossa lies:**
   A. Above the roots of canines
   B. Below the roots of canines
   C. Above the roots of premolars
   D. Below the roots of premolars

7. **Which of the following teeth has maximum sensory receptors?**
   A. Maxillary permanent first molar
   B. Mandibular permanent first molar
   C. Mandibular permanent canine
   D. Maxillary permanent canine

ANSWERS

1. **D.**   Canines are the longest teeth in the mouth.
   Tooth   *Length*
   Maxillary canine   –   27 mm
   Mandibular canine –   27 mm
   Maxillary canine has longest root and mandibular canine has longest crown.

2. **D.**   Refer to answer No. 1

3. **B.**
Tooth (Permanent)		*Mesiodistal width at crown*
Maxillary central incisor	–	8.5 mm
Maxillary lateral incisor	–	6.5 mm
Maxillary canine	–	7.5 mm
Mandibular central incisor	–	5.0 mm
Mandibular lateral incisor	–	5.5 mm
Mandibular canine	–	7 mm

4. **C.**   The root of the maxillary canine is usually the longest of any root.

5. **A.**   The cervicoincisal lengths of permanent mandibular canine and permanent maxillary canines are 11 mm and 10 mm respectively.

6. **C.**   Anterior to the canine eminence, overlying the roots of the incisor teeth, is a shallow concavity known as the incisive fossa. Posterior to the canine eminence on a higher level is a deeper concavity called the canine fossa. The floor of this canine fossa is formed in part by the projecting zygomatic process.

7. **D.**   Maxillary canines are perhaps the most disease resistant and stable because of the labiolingual thickness of crown and root and the strong anchorage in the jaws. The length of the maxillary canine is longest of all the teeth. The labiolingual dimensions of canine are the largest among all anterior teeth. Since the tooth is longer and bulky, it may also show the largest pulp chamber in the anterior teeth.

 # Maxillary Premolars

1. **When viewed from buccal aspect, the maxillary premolars resemble?**
   A. Permanent maxillary first molar
   B. Permanent maxillary canine
   C. Permanent maxillary central incisor
   D. None of the above

2. **When maxillary premolars have two roots they are placed?**
   A. One mesially and other distally
   B. One buccally and other lingually
   C. Both roots are placed lingually
   D. None of the above

3. **The maxillary first premolar has two cusps, a buccal and a lingual. Which statement is true about maxillary first premolar cusps?**
   A. The buccal cusp is about 1 mm longer than lingual cusp
   B. The lingual cusp is about 1 mm longer than buccal cusp
   C. Both the lingual and buccal cusps are of same height
   D. None of the above statements is correct

4. **The maxillary first premolar has which of the following characteristics for differentiation from other anterior teeth?**
   A. Greater relative faciolingual measurement as compared with the mesiodistal measurement
   B. Broader contact area
   C. Both contact areas are more nearly at the same level
   D. All of the above

5. **When viewed from buccal aspect the form of the maxillary first premolar is:**
   A. Rhomboidal
   B. Trapezoidal
   C. Rectangular
   D. Oval

6. **The occlusal aspect of the maxillary first premolar roughly resembles which geometric form?**
   A. Six sided or hexagonal
   B. Triangular
   C. Trapezoidal
   D. Rectangular

7. **Which premolar of the dental arch has mostly two roots ?**
   A. Mandibular first premolar
   B. Maxillary first premolar
   C. Mandibular second premolar
   D. Maxillary second premolar

ANSWERS

1. **B.** The middle labial lobe of maxillary premolars and middle lobe of maxillary canines are highly developed.

   Labial crown outline is roughly pentagon.

2. **B.** In maxillary teeth proceeding archwise mesiodistally the midline of the arch lies at the mesial corner of the second premolars.

3. **A.** The buccal cusp of maxillary first premolar assists the canine as a prehensile or tearing tooth.

4. **D.** Maxillary anterior teeth crowns are longer on an average by 2 mm than the maxillary premolar crowns. The roots of the maxillary premolars are almost equal in length to the roots of the maxillary lateral incisors but shorter than the roots of the maxillary central incisors by 1 mm and canine by 2.5 to 3 mm.

5. **B.** Maxillary first premolar resembles the canine from buccal aspect. Mesial slope of the buccal cusp is longer than the distal slope

6. **A.** The mesial side of maxillary first premolar is shorter than distal side and also the mesiolingual side is shorter than distolingual side.

7. **B.** A distinguishing feature of maxillary first premolar is found on the mesial surface of the crown, immediately cervical to the mesial contact area, centered on the mesial surface and bordered buccally and lingually by the mesiobuccal and mesiolingual line angles is a marked depression called the mesial developmental depression, which continues apically beyond the cervical line, joins a deep developmental depression between the roots and at the root bifurcation.

12 Mandibular Premolars

1. **Which characteristic(s) of mandibular first premolar resembles those of the permanent mandibular canine?**
   A. The buccal cusp is long and sharp and is the only occluding cusp
   B. The buccolingual measurement is similar to that of canine
   C. The occlusal surface slopes sharply lingually in a cervical direction
   D. All of the above

2. **Which characteristic(s) of mandibular first premolar resemble(s) those of the second mandibular premolar?**
   A. The contact areas, mesially and distally are nearly at the same level
   B. The curvature of cervical line mesially and distally is similar
   C. The tooth has more than one cusp
   D. All of the above

3. **Normally the mandibular second premolar has 3 cusps. Arrange the size of the cusp from largest to smallest:**
   A. Buccal cusp - Mesiolingual cusp - Distolingual cusp
   B. Buccal cusp - Distolingual cusp - Mesiolingual cusp
   C. Mesiolingual cusp - Distolingual cusp - Buccal cusp
   D. All the cusps have same size

4. **Which of the following permanent posterior teeth has 'Y'shaped groove on the occlusal surface?**
   A. Permanent mandibular first molar
   B. Permanent maxillary first molar
   C. Permanent mandibular second premolar
   D. Permanent maxillary second premolar

ANSWERS

1. **D.** Buccal and occlusal outline forms of mandibular first premolar resemble to mandibular canine.

2. **D.** Lingual cusp of mandibular first premolar is almost non-functional.

3. **A.** Three cusps type mandibular second premolar appears more angular from occlusal aspect than the two cusps type which is more rounded from occlusal aspect.

4. **C.** Three cusps type mandibular second premolar has Y-shaped pattern of groove on occlusal surface.

13 Permanent Maxillary Molars

1. The permanent maxillary molar has three roots. What is the arrangement of these roots?
   A. Two lingual and one buccal root
   B. Two buccal and one lingual root
   C. One mesial, one distal and one lingual root
   D. None of the above

2. Which of the following roots is the largest in permanent maxillary molar?
   A. Buccal root
   B. Lingual root
   C. Mesiobuccal root
   D. Distobuccal root

3. Which statement is *correct* about permanent maxillary first molar?
   A. Crown is wider buccolingually than mesiodistally
   B. Crown is wider mesiodistally than buccolingually
   C. Crown is equal buccolingually than mesiodistally
   D. None of the above statements is correct

4. Sometimes tubercle of Carabelli is found in permanent maxillary first molar. What is the position of the tubercle of Carabelli?
   A. Lingual to mesiolingual cusp
   B. Buccal to mesiolingual cusp
   C. Lingual to distolingual cusp
   D. Buccal to distolingual cusp

5. Which of the followings is the smallest root in permanent maxillary first molar?
   A. All the roots have same length
   B. Palatal root
   C. Mesiobuccal root
   D. Distobuccal root

6. Which of the following cusps is the largest in the permanent maxillary first molar?
   A. Mesiolingual
   B. Mesiobuccal
   C. Distolingual
   D. Distobuccal

7. The oblique ridge is found in permanent maxillary first molar that crosses the occlusal surface obliquely. It is formed by the union of:
   A. Triangular ridge of distobuccal cusp and distal ridge of mesiolingual cusp
   B. Triangular ridge of mesiobuccal cusp and distal ridge of mesiolingual cusp
   C. Triangular ridge of distolingual cusp and distal ridge of mesiolingual cusp
   D. None of the above

8. When we observe from buccal aspect, in permanent mandibular first molar, the point of furcation of the two roots is located approximately:
   A. 3 mm below the cervical line
   B. 4 mm below the cervical line
   C. 5 mm below the cervical line
   D. 2 mm below the cervical line

9. When we see from the buccal aspect in permanent maxillary first molar, the point of furcation of the two buccal roots is located approximately?
   A. 2 mm above the cervical line
   B. 5 mm above the cervical line
   C. 3 mm above the cervical line
   D. 4 mm above the cervical line

ANSWERS

1. **B.** In permanent maxillary first molar, palatal root is the longest and distobuccal root is the shortest.

2. **B.** Refer to answer No. 1

3. **A.** The crowns of maxillary and mandibular molars are wider mesiodistally than cervico-occlusal length.

4. **A.** It is a supplemental cusp of little practical use. It serves to identify the maxillary first molar.

5. **D.** Refer to answer No. 1

6. **A.** The mesiolingual cusp of permanent maxillary first molar is the largest cusp, it is followed in point of size by the mesiobuccal, distolingual, distobuccal and fifth cusp.

7. **A.** The oblique ridge is reduced in height in the center of the occlusal surface, being about on a level with the marginal ridges of the occlusal surface.

8. **A.** There is a deep developmental depression buccally on root trank of permanent mandibular first molar, which starts at the bifurcation and progresses cervically becoming more shallow unit; it terminates at or immediately above the cervical line. This depression is smooth with no developmental groove or fold.

9. **D.** *Tooth*   *Furcation distance from the cervical line*

   1. Permanent maxillary first molar
       Mesial bifircation   – 3 mm above the cervical line
       Buccal bifurcation   – 4 mm above the cervical line
       Distal bifurcation   – 5 mm or more above the cervical line
   2. Permanent mandibular first molar
       Buccal bifurcation   – 3 mm below the cervical line
       Lingual bifurcation   – 4 mm below the cervical line

 **Pulp Cavities of the Teeth**

1. **Which of the following statements is incorrect about permanent mandibular first molar?**
   A. It has two roots, one mesial and one distal
   B. It has two canals, one mesial and one distal
   C. It has three canals, mesiobuccal, mesiolingual and distal
   D. It has 5 cusps

2. **The functions of dental pulp is/are:**
   A. Formative
   B. Sensory
   C. Defensive
   D. All of the above

3. **The primary function of dental pulp is:**
   A. Dentin formation
   B. Enamel formation
   C. Cementum formation
   D. Bone formation

4. **Which of the following tooth mostly shows kidney shaped outline form in cervical cross section?**
   A. Mandibular first premolar
   B. Mandibular second premolar
   C. Maxillary first premolar
   D. Maxillary second premolar

5. **Sometimes in permanent maxillary first molar, fourth accessory canal is located in:**
   A. Mesiobuccal root
   B. Distobuccal root
   C. Palatal root
   D. None of the above

6. **Which of the following statements is *correct* about permanent mandibular central incisor?**
   A. It is the smallest tooth in the mouth
   B. Tooth usually has one canal
   C. Occasionally, two canals may be found
   D. All of the above

ANSWERS

1. **B.** Mesial root at permanent mandibualar first molar has two root canals—mesiobuccal and mesiolingual.

2. **D.** The complex sensory system within the dental pulp controls the blood flow and is responsible for at least mediation of the sensation of pain.

3. **A.** The formation of reparative or irritation dentine is a defensive response to any form of irritation, whether it be mechanical, thermal, chemical or bacterial in nature.

4. **C.** A mesial developmental groove is usually present, giving maxillary first premolar its classic indentation.

5. **A.** If an accessory mesiobuccal canal is present in permanent maxillary first molar, it will be located lingual to the mesiobuccal canal or distolingually.

6. **D.** The labiolingual dimension of permanent mandibular central incisor is very large.

15

Basic Concept of Occlusion and Malocclusion

1. **If angle of mandible is obtuse, it means that the bone belongs to:**
   A. Adult male
   B. Adult female
   C. Young female
   D. Elderly person

2. **The teeth in occlusion should have:**
   A. Surface contact
   B. Cusp fossa-relation
   C. Cusp ridges-relation
   D. Ridge sulcus apposition

3. **Bennett movement is present on:**
   A. Working side
   B. Balancing side
   C. On protusion
   D. None of the above

4. **The total contact points in occlusion are:**
   A. 136
   B. 138
   C. 142
   D. 156

5. **In canine guided occlusion, posterior teeth contact in:**
   A. Both centric and eccentric movement
   B. Only centric occlusion
   C. Only eccentric movements
   D. All of the above

6. **The tooth having maximum faciolingual inclination is:**
   A. Maxillary central incisor
   B. Maxillary canine
   C. Maxillary lateral incisor
   D. Mandibular central incisor

7. **The tooth having maximum mesiodistal angulation is:**
   A. Maxillary lateral incisor
   B. Maxillary canine
   C. Maxillary first premolar
   D. Mandibular canine

8. **The tooth having least faciolingual inclination is:**
   A. Maxillary central incisor
   B. Mandibular central incisor
   C. Maxillary first premolar
   D. Mandibular first premolar

9. **The tooth having least mesiodistal angulation is:**
   A. Mandibular central incisor
   B. Mandibular lateral incisor
   C. Mandibular molar
   D. None of the above

10. **In centric occlusion, lingual cusp of mandibular first premolar contacts:**
    A. Distal marginal ridge of maxillary canine
    B. Cingulum of maxillary canine
    C. Mesial marginal ridge of maxillary canine
    D. No part of any maxillary tooth

11. **In Thielemann's formula for balanced occlusion, which of the following *is NOT* included?**
    A. Plane of occlusion
    B. Curve of Spee
    C. Curve of Monson
    D. Condylar guidance

12. **The length of each arm of Bonwill equilateral triangle is:**
    A. 4 inches
    B. 3 inches
    C. 6 inches
    D. 3.5 inches

13. **Overjet:**
    A. Is vertical overlap between the teeth
    B. Is horizontal overlap between the teeth
    C. Cannot be changed by dentist
    D. Determines condylar guidance

14. Compared to mandibular arch, maxillary arch is:
    A. Narrow
    B. Broad
    C. Of same width
    D. None of the above

15. During protrusion maxillary central incisor occludes with mandibular:
    A. Central incisor only
    B. Lateral incisor only
    C. Central incisor and lateral incisor
    D. Both the central incisors

16. The protrusive relation places the mandibular arch forward to the maxillary arch in most cases by:
    A. 0 to 1 mm
    B. 1 to 2 mm
    C. 2 to 3 mm
    D. 3 to 4 mm

17. During lateral movements, the balancing condyle moves:
    A. Forward, downward, mesially
    B. Forward, downward, distally
    C. Backwards, downwards, mesially
    D. Forwards, upwards mesially

18. The arch form formed by centroids is:
    A. Elliptical   B. Parabolic
    C. V-shaped   D. Circular

19. In centric occlusion, the distobuccal cusp of mandibular first molar falls into:
    A. Central fossa of maxillary first molar
    B. Embrasure between first and second molar
    C. Distal fossa of maxillary first molar
    D. Central fossa of maxillary second molar

20. In centric occlusion, mesiolingual cusp of maxillary first molar falls in the:
    A. Distal fossa of mandibular first molar
    B. Central fossa of mandibular first molar
    C. Mesial triangular fossa of first molar
    D. None of the above

21. Which of the following is *untrue* about mandible?
    A. Largest bone of face
    B. Second bone to ossify
    C. Shows only intra-membranous ossification
    D. Two halves joined at symphysis menti

22. All of the following teeth have positive contact relation mesially and distally *except:*
    A. Maxillary first molar
    B. Mandibular first molar
    C. Maxillary second molar
    D. Mandibular third molar

23. The formula of balanced occlusion was given in 1938 by:
    A. Angle
    B. Von spee
    C. Monson
    D. Thielemann

24. Which of the following is *correct* formula for balanced occlusion?

    A. $\dfrac{CG.CS}{IG.CH.PO}$ CG = Condylar guidance

    B. $\dfrac{CG.IG}{CS.CH.PO}$ IG = Incisal guidance

    C. $\dfrac{CS.IG}{CG.CH.PO}$ CS = Curve of spee

    D. $\dfrac{CG.IG.CS}{CH.PO}$ CH = Cusp height

    PO = Plane of occlusion

25. On an average how many times the closure of the jaw occurs in a single day to facilitate swallowing?
    A. 300 times
    B. 400 times
    C. 500 times
    D. 600 times

ANSWERS

1. **D.**

2. **A.** These contacting occlusal surfaces are found at incisal portions of mandibular anterior which contact with the lingual surfaces of maxillary anterior teeth.

3. **A.** In lateral movements the condyle appears to rotate with a slight lateral shift in the direction of the movement, called Bennett movement.

4. **B.** Hellman listed 138 points of possible occlusal contacts.

5. **B.** It is also called as anterior guidance, which refers to tooth guidance for all or any of the anterior teeth or to guidance involving the neuromuscular system.

6. **A.** For maximum stability and efficiency, each tooth must be placed at such an angulation so that it can best withstand the forces acting on it during functions.

7. **B.** Refer to answer No. 6

8. **C.** Refer to answer No. 6

9. **B.** Refer to answer No. 6

10. **D.** First mandibular premolar occluds partly with the maxillary first premolar and partly with the maxillary canine.

11. **C.** The Thielemann's formula for balanced occlusion is:

$$\text{Balance} = \frac{CG \times IG}{CS \times CH \times PO}$$

where,

CG= Condylar guidance, CS= Curve of Spee, CH= Cusp height, IG =Incisal guidance and PO= Plane of occlusion.

12. **A.** Bonwill has described the mandibular arch as adapting itself in part of an equilateral triangle of 4 inches.

13. **B.** The significance of overjet and overbite has to be related to the type and degree of jaw movement possible in

humans. The degree of overjet and overbite should be sufficient to allow jaw movement in function without interference.

14. B.   This relation is brought about by the differences in mesiodistal width between maxillary and mandibular anterior teeth (particularly the incisors) and by the lingual projection of mandibular posterior tooth crowns, an arrangement that brings about proper intercuspation.

15. C.   During the protrusive movement, the mandible is depressed, then moves directly forward, bringing the anterior teeth together at points most favourable for the incision of food.

16. B.   In normal functional protrusive movements, the mandibular arch is 1 to 2 mm forward than the maxillary arch.

17. A.   The condyle opposite to the side of movement is called as balancing condyle.

18. B.

19. A.   The mesiolingual cusp of the maxillary first molar makes contact with the central fossa of the mandibular first molar in centric occlusion.

20. B.   Refer to answer No. 19

21. C.   Mandibular body forms from intramembranous ossification and mandibular condyle from intrachondral ossification.

22. D.   Mandibular third molar is the last tooth in the arch.

23. D.   Refer to answer No. 11

24. B.   Refer to answer No. 11

25. D.   Swallowing involves most of the tongue muscles and buccal musculature.

16 Dento-osseous Structures

1. **Angle of the mandible is everted in:**
   A. Males
   B. Females
   C. Both
   D. None of the above

2. **Mental foramen is located near the lower border of mandible at:**
   A. Birth
   B. In adults
   C. Old age
   D. None of the above

3. **Bite marks caused by premolar have:**
   A. Rectangular shape
   B. Two point diamond shape
   C. Triangular shape
   D. No characteristic shape

4. **The largest bone in face is:**
   A. Maxilla
   B. Mandible
   C. Zygomatic
   D. Frontal

5. **The right and left halves of mandible fuse at:**
   A. Symphysis menti
   B. Incisive fossa
   C. Mental protuberance
   D. Genial tubercles

6. **Most often, the mental foramen is located:**
   A. Below first premolar
   B. Between first and second premolar
   C. Below second premolar
   D. None of the above

7. **The mental foramen is directed:**
   A. Downward, forward, laterally
   B. Upward, forward, laterally
   C. Downward, backward, laterally
   D. Upward, backward and laterally

8. **In childhood, mental foramen is located:**
   A. Below first primary molar
   B. Below second primary molar
   C. Between first and second primary molars
   D. None of the above

9. **The mylohyoid line gives origin to which muscle?**
   A. Anterior belly of digastric
   B. Platysma
   C. Mylohyoid
   D. Superior constrictor

10. **The opening of mandibular canal on the medial side of mandible is marked by a bony projection called:**
    A. Lingula
    B. Pterygoid fossa
    C. Genial tubercles
    D. None of the above

11. **The ligament attached to lingula is:**
    A. Stylomandibular
    B. Sphenomandibular
    C. Temporomandibular
    D. None of the above

12. **The muscle inserted on pterygoid fovea is:**
    A. Medial pterygoid
    B. Lateral pterygoid
    C. Temporalis
    D. Superior constrictor

13. **"Antrum of Highmore" is another name of:**
    A. Sphenoid sinus
    B. Frontal sinus
    C. Maxillary sinus
    D. Ethmoidal sinus

14. **The largest of all paranasal sinuses is:**
    A. Frontal
    B. Sphenoid
    C. Ethmoid
    D. Maxillary

15. **The capacity of a full grown maxillary sinus is:**
    A. 3-5 ml
    B. 7-10 ml
    C. 10-15 ml
    D. 20-30 ml

16. **The roof of maxillary sinus is formed by:**
    A. Nasoantral wall
    B. Orbital plate of maxilla
    C. Alveolar process
    D. Sphenomaxillary wall

17. **Out of the following, which of the processes does not belong to maxilla?**
    A. Palatine
    B. Alveolar
    C. Zygomatic
    D. Temporal

18. **Maxilla articulates with the following bone(s):**
    A. Lacrimal
    B. Ethmoid
    C. Frontal
    D. All of the above

19. **Hard palate is formed by:**
    A. Palatine process of maxilla
    B. Horizontal plate of palatine bone
    C. Both of the above
    D. Neither of the above

20. **Midline foramina of incisive canal is called:**
    A. Foramen of Scarpa
    B. Foramen of Larschak
    C. Foramen of Stenson
    D. Foramen Rotundum

21. **Medial surface of mandible has all of the followings** *except*:
    A. Lingula
    B. Submandibular foramen
    C. Mental foramen
    D. Mandibular foramen

22. **Sutures present in palate are:**
    A. Intermaxillary
    B. Interpalatine
    C. Palatomaxillary
    D. All of the above

23. **Upper genial tubercles give origin to:**
    A. Genioglossus
    B. Geniohyoid
    C. Anterior belly of digastric
    D. Pterygomandibular raphe

24. **Which statement is** *correct* **about maxillary sinus?**
    A. Pyramidal in shape, base is directed to nasal cavity
    B. Hexagonal in shape, base is directed to nasal cavity
    C. Oval shape, apex is divided to nasal cavity
    D. Pyramidal shape, apex is directed to nasal cavity

25. **The sensory nerve supply to the jaws and teeth is derived from:**
    A. Fourth cranial nerve
    B. Fifth cranial nerve
    C. Seventh cranial nerve
    D. Ninth cranial nerve

26. **The mandibular nerve leaves the skull through the:**
    A. Foramen ovale
    B. Foramen rotundum
    C. Foramen spinosum
    D. Foramen magnum

27. **Which muscle is supplied by mylohyoid nerve?**
    A. Only mylohyoid muscle
    B. Mylohyoid muscle and anterior belly of digastric muscle
    C. Mylohyoid muscle and posterior belly of digastric muscle
    D. Only digastric muscle

28. **Lower lip and chin are supplied by the:**
    A. Mylohyoid nerve
    B. Facial nerve
    C. Mental nerve
    D. All of the above

29. **Mental foramen is *NOT* located near the lower border of mandible at:**
    A. Birth
    B. In adults
    C. Both the above
    D. None of the above

30. **Which of the following facial bones *does not* have an osseous union with skull?**
    A. Maxillae
    B. Mandible
    C. Zygomatic
    D. Frontal process of maxillae

31. **Which is *NOT* the maxillary "surface"?**
    A. Orbital surface
    B. Infratemporal surface
    C. Facial surface
    D. None of the above

32. **Floor of the orbit is formed by:**
    A. Orbital surface of maxilla
    B. Orbital surface of zygomatic bone
    C. Both (A) and (B)
    D. None of the above

33. **"Lacrimal groove" is a notch present on:**
    A. Medial edge of orbital surface
    B. Medial edge of ethmoid bone
    C. Medial edge of nasal bone
    D. Frontal bone

34. **'Foramina of Stensen opens into:**
    A. Incisive fossa
    B. Incisive foramen
    C. Mandibular canal
    D. Incisive canal

35. **Foramina of Stensen carries which of the following structures?**
    A. Nasopalatine nerves and vessels
    B. Olfactory nerves
    C. Greater palatine nerve
    D. None of the above

36. **Foramina of Scarpa is present on:**
    A. Maxillary third molar region
    B. Mandibular incisor region
    C. Maxillary incisor region
    D. None of the above

37. **Inferior portion of maxilla is formed by:**
    A. Palatine process   B. Zygomatic process
    C. Alveolar process   D. Frontal process

38. **Which of the following statements about maxillary alveolar process is/are *true*?**
    A. Facial plate is thin
    B. Lingually bone is very thick
    C. Lingual plate of alveolar process is heavier than the facial plate
    D. All of the above

39. **Generally, maxillary lingual plate is heavier, however lingual plate is 'paper thin' over:**
    A. Third molar alveolus
    B. First molar alveolus
    C. Canine
    D. None of the above

40. **Thin maxillary lingual plate is thin over molar roots due to:**
    A. Formation of greater palatine canal
    B. Formation of incisive foramen
    C. Greater palatine foramen
    D. None of the above

41. **Alveolar process is maintained by:**
    A. Presence of teeth
    B. Absence of teeth
    C. Is not affected by teeth
    D. Does not reduce after tooth loss

42. **'Kidney shaped' alveolus is found with:**
    A. Maxillary first premolar
    B. Maxillary second premolar
    C. Mesial root of mandibular first molar
    D. All of the above

43. **The alveolus of which tooth is "triangular" in cross section with apex towards lingual side?**
    A. Mandibular central incisor
    B. Mandibular canine
    C. Maxillary central incisor
    D. Maxillary canine

44. **Second alveolus from median line is lateral incisor which is:**
    A. Round
    B. Kidney shaped
    C. Conical and egg shaped
    D. None of the above

45. **Alveolar process is:**
    A. The portion of the jaw which serves as a support for the tooth
    B. The bone of the tooth socket
    C. Both of the above
    D. None of the above

ANSWERS

1. **A.**

2. **A.** Mental foramen is directed upward and backward as well as laterally.

3. **B.**

4. **B.** The single, horseshoe-shaped mandible is the largest and strongest bone of the face and forms a framework for the floor of the month.

5. **A.** Symphysis menti is a faint ridge in the middle of the mandible.

6. **C.** Mental foramen forms the anterior opening of the mandibular canal. Its position is not constant.

7. **D.** Refer to answer No. 2

8. **A.** In childhood, mental foramen is also near the lower border of the mandible.

9. **C.** The mylohyoid line running forwards and downward on each side from the third molar tooth to the symphysis menti divides the internal surface into two areas – submandibular fossa below the line, and sublingual fossa above the line.

10. **A.** Lingula or mandibular spine gives attachment to the spheno mandibular ligament.

11. **B.** Refer to answer No. 10

12. **B.** The neck of the condyle is a constricted portion immediately below the articular surfaces. It is flattened in front and presents a concave pit medially –the pterygoid fovea.

13. **C.** Maxillary sinus presents as a small cavity at birth, starting its development during the third fetal month and it reaches its maximum development by about the eighteenth year of life. It is the longest of all sinuses.

14. **D.** Refer to answer No. 13

15. **C.** At the age of eighteen, the capacity of the maxillary sinus is about 10 to 15 ml or about 1 tablespoon. The average size of the maxillary sinus in an adult is 25 mm transversely, 30 mm anteroposteriorly, and 30 mm vertically.

16. **B.** Shape of the maxillary sinus is similar to four-sided pyramid. The base of the pyramid is directed medially towards the lateral wall of the nose. The apex is directed laterally in the zygomatiz process of the maxilla.

17. **D.** Temporal bone is a separate bone of the skull. All other are parts of maxilla.

18. **D.** The maxilla articulates with the nasal, frontal, lacrimal and ethmoid bones above, and laterally with the zygomatic bone, and occasionally with the sphenoid bone.

19. **C.** Palatine processes form the anterior three fourths of the hard palate as far posteriorly as the second molar where they articulate with the horizontal parts of the palatine bone, and thus forms a greater part of the roof of the oral cavity and floor of the nasal cavity.

20. **A.** Incisive fossa into which the incisive canals open may be seen immediately lingual to the maxillary central incisors at the median line, or intermaxillary suture when the maxilla are joined. Two canals open laterally into the incisive foramen, the foramina of Stenson, carrying the nasopalatine nerves and vessels. Occasionally, two midline foramina are present, the foramina of scarpi.

21. **C.** Mental foramen is present on the external surface at the body of the mandible.

22. **D.** Maxilla consists of a body and four processes: the zygomatic, frontal, palatine and alveolar processes.

23. **A.** Inferior genial tubercles or mental spines give origin to geniohyoid muscles.

24. **A.** The maxillary sinus overlies the alveolar process in which the molar teeth are implanted, more particularly

the first and second molars, the alveoli of which are separated from the sinus by a thin layer of bone.

25. **B.** It is called trigeminal nerve.

26. **A.** After leaving the skull through the foramen ovale, the mandibular nerve almost immediately breaks up into its several branches.

27. **B.** Mylohyoid nerve is the motor branch of mandibular nerve.

28. **C.** Mental nerve is the branch of mandibular nerve.

29. **C.** The mental foramen is usually located midway between the superior and inferior border of the body of the mandible when the teeth are in position, and most often it is below the second premolar tooth, a little below the apex of the root. After the teeth are lost and resorption of alveolar bone has taken place, the mental foramen may appear near the crest of the alveolar bone.

30. **B.** The mandible is movable and is situated immediately below the maxillary and zygomatic bone, and its condyles rest in the mandibular fossa of the temporal bone. This articulation is called temporomandibular joint or TMJ.

31. **D.** Facial surface is also called anterior surface and infratemporal surface is also called posterior surface. Orbital surface is smooth and together with the orbital surface of the zygomatic bone forms the floor of the orbit.

32. **C.** Refer to answer No. 31

33. **A.** Traversing the posterior portion of the orbital surface is the infraorbital groove.

34. **B.** Two canals open laterally into the incisive foramen, the foramina of Stenson, carrying the nasopalatine nerves and vessels.

35. **A.** Refer to answer No. 34

36. **C.** These are the midline foramina.

37. **C.** The facial plate of maxillary alveolar process is thin. The buccal plate over the second and third molars, including the alveolar margins, is thicker. Generally, the lingual plate of the maxillary alveolar process is heavier than the facial plate

38. **D.** Refer to answer No. 37

39. **B.** This thin lingual plate over the molar tooth is part of the formation of the greater palatine canal.

40. **A.** Refer to answer No. 39

41. **A.** Should any tooth be lost, that portion of the alveolar process which support the missing tooth will be subject to atrophic reduction. Should all of the teeth be lost, the alveolar process will eventually cease to exits.

42. **D.** The maxillary first premolar alveolus is kidney-shaped in cross-section with the cavity partially divided by a spine of bone, which fits into the mesial developmental groove of the root of this tooth. The maxillary second premolar–alveolar is also kidney-shaped, but the curvatures are in reverse to those of the first premolar alveolus. The septal spine is located on the distal side instead of the mesial.

    The alveolus of mesial root of permanent mandibular first molar is much wider buccolingually than mesiodistally, and constricted in the center to accommodate developmental grooves found mesial and distal to the mesial root.

43. **C.** The cross section of maxillary central incisor is triangular in shape with apex located lingually.

44. **C.** Alveolus of maxillary lateral incisor is conical and egg-shaped or ovoid and that of mandibular lateral incisor is flattened on its mesial surface.

45. **C.** Alveolar process is made up of labiobuccal and lingual plates of very dense but thin cortical bone separated by interdental septa of cancellous bone.

Temporomandibular Joints and their Functions

1. **The head of condylar process of mandible is covered by:**
   A. Hyaline cartilage
   B. Loose connective tissue
   C. Fibrocartilage
   D. Loose areolar tissue

2. **Glenoid fossa is:**
   A. Depression in the temporal bone in which mandibular condyle articulates
   B. Another name for mandibular notch
   C. Another name for central fossa
   D. Attachment of temporalis muscle

3. **The long axis of mandibular condyle is directed:**
   A. Anteromedially
   B. Anterolaterally
   C. Posteromedially
   D. Posterolaterally

4. **The temporomandibular joint is a:**
   A. Diarthrosis
   B. Monoarthrosis
   C. Both of the above
   D. None of the above

5. **The movement of temporomandibular joint is:**
   A. Only Gliding movement
   B. Only Hinge movement
   C. Both Gliding movement and Hinge movement
   D. None of the above

6. **In TMJ, the central area of articular disc is:**
   A. Avascular and devoid of nerve
   B. Vascular and devoid of nerve
   C. Avascular and contains nerve
   D. None of the above

7. **In TMJ, there are upper and lower compartments. Which of the following statement(s) is *correct* about this?**
   A. Upper compartment shows gliding movement and lower compartment shows hinge movement
   B. Upper compartment shows hinge movement and lower compartment shows gliding movement
   C. Both compartments show only hinge movement
   D. Both the compartments show only gliding movement

8. **The Bennett movement is:**
   A. Protrusive movement
   B. Retrusive movement
   C. Medial movement
   D. Lateral movement

9. **Which of the following statement(s) is/are *correct* about lateral pterygoid muscle?**
   A. Superior head has a closing movement
   B. Inferior head has an opening movement
   C. The insertion is on the anterior surface of the neck of condyle
   D. All of the above

10. **Which function is not performed by lateral pterygoid muscle?**
    A. Protrusion of mandible
    B. Depression of mandible
    C. Lateral movement of mandible
    D. Grinding and retrusion

11. **Which muscle of face is affected by emotions and is active in facial expression ?**
    A. Temporalis   B. Masseter
    C. Lateral pterygoid   D. Risorius

12. **Which muscle is a synergist for the lateral pterygoid muscle?**
    A. Masseter   B. Buccinator
    C. Lateral pterygoid   D. Medial pterygoid

13. **The origin of the medial pterygoid muscle is:**
    A. Medial surface of the lateral pterygoid plate
    B. Medial surface of the medial pterygoid plate
    C. Lateral surface of the lateral pterygoid plate
    D. Lateral surface of the medial pterygoid plate

14. **The principal function of the medial pterygoid muscle is:**
    A. Protrusion of mandible
    B. Elevation of mandible
    C. Lateral positioning of the mandible
    D. All of the above

15. **The shape of the temporalis muscle is:**
    A. Fan-shaped   B. Funnel-shaped
    C. Pear-shaped   D. Heart-shaped

16. **The digastric muscle is supplied by the:**
    A. Mandibular nerve
    B. Facial nerve
    C. Both mandibular and facial nerves
    D. None of the above

17. **Which of the following statements is/are *correct* about the geniohyoid muscle?**
    A. It arises from the mental spine on the posterior aspect of the symphysis menti
    B. It inserts on the anterior surface of the hyoid bone
    C. It is supplied by C_1, C_2 and hypoglossal nerve
    D. All of the above

18. **Which of the following muscles *does not* function as a depressor of mandible?**
    A. Digastric
    B. Mylohyoid
    C. Geniohyoid
    D. Temporalis

19. **Elevation against resistance is affected by the:**
    A. Temporalis muscle
    B. Masseter muscle
    C. Medial pterygoid muscle
    D. All of the above

20. **The muscles of facial expression are innervated by the:**
    A. 5th cranial nerve
    B. 7th cranial nerve
    C. 9th cranial nerve
    D. 11th cranial nerve

ANSWERS

1. **C.** The fibrous layers of the temporomandibular joint are avascular.

2. **A.** Glenoid fossa is also called the mandibular fossa.

3. **C.** The long axes of the condyles are in lateral plane, If the lines were prolonged, The long axes would meet at a point anterior to the foramen magnum at an angle of approximately 135 degree.

4. **A.** The osseous portions of the TMJ are the anterior portion of the mandibular (glenoid) fossa and articular eminence of the temporal bone and the condyloid process of the mandible.

5. **C.** The articular space is divided into upper and lower compartments by the articular disk. The rotational movements occur in the lower joint space, while the sliding movements occur in the upper joint space.

6. **A.** Articular disc consists of dense collagenous connective tissue, which, in the central area, is relatively avascular, hyalinized and devoid of nerves. The disc is not seen on radiographs, but the bony structures of TMJ in one plane can be viewed by a transcranial projection.

7. **A.** Refer to answer No. 5

8. **D.** In lateral movements, the condyle appears to rotate with a slight lateral shift in the direction of the movement called Bennett movement and may have immediate as well as progressive components.

9. **D.** Lateral pterygoid muscle has two heads of origin, upper or superior head originates on the greater sphenoid wing. Inferior head originates on the outer surface of the lateral pterygoid plate.

10. **D.** Temporal muscle is the principle positioner of the mandible during elevation. The posterior part is active in retruding the mandible and the anterior part is active during clenching.

11. **D.** Risorius is the muscle of facial expression.

12. **A.** Masseter muscle may also be an antagonist to the posterior temporalis.

13. **A.** It also originates from the palatine bone.

14. **D.** Medial pterygoid muscle is inserted on the medial surface of the angle of mandible and on the ramus upto the mandibular foramen.

15. **A.** Temporal muscle originates in the temporal fossa.

16. **C.** Mylohyoid branch of the mandibular division of the fifth nerve innervates the anterior digastric muscle; the digastric branch of the facial nerve innervates the posterior digastric muscle.

17. **D.** When the hyoid bone is fixed, geniohyoid depresses the mandible and when the lower jaw is fixed, it moves the hyoid bone forward and upward.

18. **D.** Actions of temporal muscles are as follows:
    i. Principal positioner of the mandible during elevation.
    ii. Posterior part retrudes the mandible.
    iii. Anterior part is synergistic with the masseter in clenching.
    iv. Posterior part acts as an antogonist to the masseter in retruding the jaw.

19. **D.** The masseter muscle is active during forceful jaw closing and may assist in protrusion of the mandible.
    Also refer answer No. 17.

20. **B.** Muscles of mastication are innervated by fifth cranial nerve.

18 Miscellaneous

1. **When is the first evidence of calcification of primary teeth?**
   A. 4 months *in utero*
   B. 4 and ½ months *in utero*
   C. 5 months *in utero*
   D. 6 months *in utero*

2. **The last primary tooth to be replaced by a permanent tooth is usually:**
   A. Maxillary canine
   B. Mandibular canine
   C. Maxillary first molar
   D. Mandibular second molar

3. **The commonest teeth involved in transposition are:**
   A. Maxillary central incisor and lateral incisor
   B. Maxillary canine and first premolar
   C. Maxillary first premolar and second premolar
   D. Maxillary canine and lateral incisor

ANSWERS

1. **A.** The enamel of the crown of deciduous teeth begins to calcify between 3 to 4 months in utero (12 to 16 weeks) and completes the calcification at about 11 months.

2. **A.** The first molars are the first teeth of permanent dentition to erupt followed by central incisors. After central incisors mandibular lateral incisor erupt which is followed by maxillary lateral incisors. The first premolars erupt after maxillary laterals and mandibular canine also at the same time or little later. After one year of manidbular canine eruption, second premolars erupt, which are followed by maxillary canine.

3. **D.** In transposition teeth are not placed at their normal places. They exchange their places with another teeth. It is mostly seen in case of maxillary canine, which erupt in place of maxillary lateral incisor and vice versa.

MCQs on Oral and
Dental Histology
and Embryology

Development and Growth of Face and Oral Cavity

1. After fertilization of ovum, series of cell divisions give rise to an egg cell mass called:
   A. Placenta   B. Morula
   C. Embryo   D. Embryonic disc

2. In humans, the major portion of the egg cell mass forms the:
   A. Extra embryonic membranes
   B. Embryo
   C. Embryonic disc
   D. Morula

3. 1/4th of the cells of the egg cell mass form a single layer which forms:
   A. Embryo
   B. Placenta
   C. Extra embryonic membrane
   D. Morula

4. A unique population of cells develop from the ectoderm along the lateral margin and are called:
   A. Neural crest cells
   B. Enamel
   C. Notochord
   D. Neural fold

5. All of the following are formed by neural crest cells *except:*
   A. Cartilage   B. Enamel
   C. Dentin   D. Bone

6. Most of the hard palate and all of the soft palate form from the:
   A. Primary palate
   B. Secondary palate
   C. Accessory palate
   D. None of the above

7. **In humans, how many visceral arches are there?**
   A. 2
   B. 4
   C. 5
   D. 6

8. **In humans, which visceral arch is rudimentary?**
   A. 2nd
   B. 4th
   C. 5th
   D. 6th

9. **The name of the first visceral arch is:**
   A. Mandibular
   B. Hyoid
   C. Maxillary
   D. None of the above

10. **Name the second visceral arch is:**
    A. Maxillary
    B. Mandibular
    C. Hyoid
    D. None of the above

11. **Which of the following statements is/are *true*?**
    A. Anterior 2/3rd of the tongue is covered by ectoderm and posterior 1/3rd is covered by endoderm
    B. Thyroid gland forms by invagination of the most anterior endoderm
    C. Foramen caecum is present at junction of anterior 2/3rd and posterior 1/3rd of the tongue
    D. All of the above

12. **Which of the following statements is/are *true*?**
    A. About 2/3rd of patients with cleft of the primary palate also have cleft of the secondary palate
    B. After cleft involving the primary palate, the second most common facial malformation in humans is cleft involving only secondary palate
    C. Hemifacial microsomia is the third most common facial malformation
    D. All of the above

13. **Treacher Collins' syndrome is:**
    A. Mandibulofacial dysostosis
    B. Maxillofacial dysostosis
    C. Deformity of hair
    D. None of the above

14. **Median rhomboid glossitis is:**
    A. Caused by persistence of tuberculum impar
    B. Red and rhomboidal smooth zone of the tongue
    C. Found in mid line in front of the foramen caecum
    D. All of the above

15. **Which drug causes malformations similar to hemifacial microsomia when taken during early pregnancy?**
    A. Thalidomide   B. Nicotinamide
    C. Procainamide   D. Vitamin D

16. **Globulomaxillary cyst is found between:**
    A. Central incisors
    B. Central incisor and lateral incisor
    C. Lateral incisor and canine
    D. Canine and premolar

17. **Every branchial arch contains which of the following structures?**
    A. Branchial artery
    B. Branchiomeric nerve
    C. Branchial arch cartilage rod
    D. All of the above

18. **The philtrum of the upper lip is formed largely by:**
    A. Maxillary processes
    B. Globular process
    C. Lateral nasal processes
    D. None of the above

19. **The nerve supply of the muscles of mastication shows that these muscles are derived from the:**
    A. Third branchial arch
    B. Fourth branchial arch
    C. First branchial arch
    D. Second branchial arch

20. **In the embryo, the upper lip is formed by the fusion of the:**
    A. Premaxilla with maxillary processes
    B. Median nasal process with lateral nasal processes
    C. First branchial arch with second branchial arch
    D. Median nasal processes with maxillary processes

21. **The primitive endoderm is formed from the:**
    A. Embryonic disc
    B. Trophoblast
    C. Amniotic cavity
    D. Primitive yolk sac

22. **The neural tube gives rise to the:**
    A. Nervous system
    B. Primitive endoderm
    C. Embryonic disc
    D. Neural groove

23. **The buccopharyngeal membrane is formed:**
    A. When the stomodeum ectoderm contacts the endoderm of the foregut
    B. From fifth branchial arch
    C. From tuberculum impar
    D. From the primitive gut

24. **A shelf-like extension of the frontonasal process separates the anterior part of the common nasal and oral cavity. The extension is termed the:**
    A. Primitive mouth
    B. Primitive palate
    C. Primitive nasal septum
    D. Stomodeum

ANSWERS

1. **B.** Morula is a solid mass of cells, resembling a mulberry.

2. **A.** Less than one-fourth of the cells of the egg cell mass eventually assemble to form a single layer which will form the embryo.

3. **A.** Refer to answer No. 2

4. **A.** Neural crest cells undergo extensive migrations, usually beginning at about the time of tube closure.

5. **B.** The neural crest cells that migrate in the trunk region form mostly neural, endocrine and pigment cells. Enamel forming cells are derived from ectoderm lining the oral cavity.

6. **B.** New outgrowths from the medial edges of the maxillary prominences form the shelves of the secondary palate.

7. **D.** Fifth arch is rudimentary.

8. **C.** Refer to answer No. 7

9. **A.** Second visceral arch is hyoid arch.

10. **C.** Myoblasts from the first arch contribute mostly to the muscles of mastication.

11. **D.** Connective tissue components of the anterior two-thirds of the tongue are derived from first–arch mesenchyme, whereas those of the posterior one-third, appear to be primarily derived from the third arch mesenchyme.

12. **D.** Clefts of the primary palate can be produced by several procedures that reduce the number of crest cells prior to migration and consequently reduce the size of the facial prominences.

13. **A.** It results from the action of dominant gene.

14. **D.** Lack of fusion between the two lateral lingual prominences may produces a bifid tongue.

15. **A.** Thalidomide and other chemical agents cause hemorrhage at the point of fusion between the external carotid and stapedial arteries.

16. **C.** It may arise from epithelial rests after the fusion of medial and lateral nasal prominences.

17. **D.** In humans there is a total of six visceral arches, of which the fifth is rudimentary.

18. **D.** From the medial nasal processes develops the philtrum.

19. **C.** The mesoderm of mandibular (first) arch gives rise to the fifth nerve and myoblast from the first arch contribute mostly to the muscles of mastication.

20. **D.** The medial and lateral nasal prominences contact each other below the developing nasal pit to form the primary palate.

21. **D.** Trophoblast forms the placenta.

22. **A.** During the third week after fertilization, neural folds appear from the lateral edges of the neural plate.

23. **A.** At about the twenty-seventh day of gestation this membrane ruptures and the primitive oral cavity establishes a connection with the foregut.

24. **B.** It forms the roof of the anterior portion of the primitive oral cavity, as well as forming the initial separation between the oral and nasal cavities.

Development of Teeth

1. **Dental lamina is formed when:**
   A. The embryo is 3 weeks old
   B. The embryo is 4 weeks old
   C. The embryo is 5 weeks old
   D. The embryo is 6 weeks old

2. **Which statement(s) is/are *true*?**
   A. The development of the first permanent molar is initiated at the 4th month of intrauterine life
   B. The second permanent molar is initiated at about the first year after birth
   C. The third molar is initiated at the 4th or 5th years after birth
   D. All of the above

3. **The successor of the deciduous teeth develops from:**
   A. Lingual extension of the dental lamina
   B. Labial extension of the dental lamina
   C. Buccal extension of the dental lamina
   D. Occlusal extension of the dental lamina

4. **The lingual extension of dental lamina is known as:**
   A. Mental lamina   B. Mandibular lamina
   C. Successional lamina   D. Maxillary lamina

5. **Life of successional lamina is from the:**
   A. 5th month *in utero* to the 10th month of age
   B. 3rd month *in utero* to the 10th month of age
   C. 5th month *in utero* to the 8th month *in utero*
   D. 6 weeks of embryo to the 8th month *in utero*

6. **Total activity of the dental lamina extends over a period of:**
   A. At least 3 years
   B. At least 4 years
   C. At least 5 years
   D. At least 6 years

7. **Epithelial pearls are:**
   A. Remnants of dental lamina
   B. Remnants of Hertwig's epithelial root sheath
   C. Remnants of diaphragm
   D. Remnants of enamel

8. **Epithelial pearls are found:**
   A. Within the jaw
   B. In the gingiva
   C. None of the above
   D. Both (A) and (B)

9. **The cells of the dental papilla will form:**
   A. Tooth pulp
   B. Dentin
   C. Both of the above
   D. None of the above

10. **The cells in the dental sac will form:**
    A. Cementum
    B. Periodontal ligament
    C. Dentin
    D. Both (A) and (B)

11. **The cells in the center of the enamel organ are densely packed and form:**
    A. The enamel knot
    B. Strips of cloth
    C. Surgical knot
    D. All of the above

12. **Which statement is *false*?**
    A. A vertical extension of the enamel knot is formed by enamel cord
    B. The function of the enamel cord and knot is to act as a reservoir of the dividing cells for the growing enamel organ
    C. The epithelial enamel organ, the dental papilla and the dental sac are the formative tissues for entire tooth and its supporting structures
    D. None of the above

13. **The size of the ameloblast cell is:**
   A. 4 to 5 microns in diameter and about 40 microns in length
   B. 6 to 8 microns in diameter and about 60 microns in length
   C. 6 to 8 microns in diameter and about 40 microns in length
   D. 1 to 2 microns in diameter and about 60 microns in length

14. **The basement membrane that separates the enamel organ and the dental papilla just prior to dentin formation is called the:**
   A. Advanced bell stage
   B. Membrana preformativa
   C. Cap stage
   D. Enamel knot

15. **Hertwig's root sheath consists of:**
   A. The outer and inner enamel epithelium only
   B. The stratum intermedium
   C. The stellate reticulum
   D. All of the above

16. **The remnants of epithelial root sheath found in periodontal ligament are called:**
   A. Enamel pearls
   B. Enamel knots
   C. Rests of Malassez
   D. Epithelial diaphragm

17. **If cells of the epithelial root sheath remain adherent to dentine surface, they may differentiate into ameloblasts and produce enamel. Such droplets of enamel are called:**
   A. Epithelial pearls
   B. Enamel pearls
   C. Rests of Malassez
   D. Epithelial diaphragm

18. **Development of accessory root canal is due to:**
   A. The broken continuity of Hertwig's root sheath
   B. The tongue-like extension of the horizontal diaphragm development
   C. The apposition of dentine and cementum to the apex of the root
   D. None of the above

19. **Which of the following statement(s) is/are *true*?**
    A. Teeth may develop in abnormal location
    B. A lack of initiation results in the absence of either single or multiple teeth
    C. A lack of initiation mostly affects the permanent upper lateral incisor, third molar and lower second premolar
    D. All of the above

20. **Which of the following statement(s) is/are *true*?**
    A. Enamel does not form in the absence of dentin
    B. In vitamin A deficiency the ameloblast fails to differentiate properly
    C. In vitamin A deficiency, atypical dentin (osteodentin) is formed
    D. All of the above

21. **Retarded eruption of teeth occurs in persons with:**
    A. Hypopituitarism and hypothyroidism
    B. Hyperpituitarism
    C. Hyperthyroidism
    D. None of the above

22. **Shape and size of teeth is determined by which stage?**
    A. Initiation   B. Histodifferentiation
    C. Morphodifferentiation D. Apposition

23. **Supernumerary teeth are formed due to abnormality in:**
    A. Initiation   B. Proliferation
    C. Histodifferentiation   D. Morphodifferentiation

24. **The final products of the embryonic dental papilla are:**
    A. Pulp, dentin and cementum only
    B. Pulp and dentin only
    C. Pulp, dentin, cementum and the periodontal ligament
    D. None of the above

25. **After formation of the deciduous tooth germ, the dental lamina:**
    A. Becomes atrophic and dormant
    B. Forms the salivary glands
    C. Degenerates
    D. Proliferates lingually to each deciduous tooth germ producing permanent tooth buds

26. The extension of the dental lamina lingual to each deciduous tooth germ is termed the:
    A. Successional dental lamina **B.** Linguoalveolar sulcus
    C. Lip furrow band   **D.** Secondary tooth bud

27. The proliferation of the dental lamina beyond the tooth germ of the second deciduous molar is the origin of the:
    A. Major salivary glands
    B. Peridens
    C. Tooth germs of the permanent molars
    D. Distomolars

28. The three permanent molars develop at:
    A. Eight months of fetal life
    B. At birth, 2½ to 3 years and 7 to 10 years after birth respectively
    C. Four months of fetal life
    D. Eight months fetal life, 3 years after birth and 6 years after birth respectively

29. Every tooth germ passes through the following stages:
    A. Dental lamina and bell stage
    B. Dental lamina, histodifferentiation and apposition of dental tissues
    C. Dental lamina and bud stage, cap stage, bell stage and apposition of dental tissues
    D. None of the above

30. The bell stage of tooth development refers to:
    A. Dental lamina
    B. Apposition of dental tissues
    C. Proliferation
    D. Histodifferentiation and morphodifferentiation

31. In the cap stage the following cell types can be recognized in the enamel organ:
    A. Outer enamel epithelium, inner enamel epithelium and stratum intermedium
    B. Outer enamel epithelium and inner enamel epithelium
    C. Stellate reticulum and dental papilla
    D. Outer enamel epithelium, inner enamel epithelium and stellate reticulum

32. **The stellate reticulum (enamel pulp) contains:**
    A. No intercellular fluid
    B. Poor quantity of mucopolysaccharide and rich amount of Tomes' fibers
    C. A large quantity of intercellular fluid
    D. A small quantity of intercellular fluid

33. **The cap stage contains the following transitory structures:**
    A. Enamel knot, enamel cord and enamel niche
    B. Enamel matrix
    C. Stratum intermedium
    D. Cervical loop

34. **The inner enamel epithelium develops into the:**
    A. Stellate reticulum   B. Ameloblasts
    C. Odontoblasts   D. Dental papilla

35. **The stratum intermedium:**
    A. Is highly gelatinous and rich in mucopolysaccharides
    B. Does not provide a reserve source of cells for the stratum intermedium
    C. Lies between the inner enamel epithelium and stellate reticulum
    D. Plays no role in enamel calcification

36. **Prior to formation of enamel matrix the stellate reticulum of the enamel organ:**
    A. Proliferates
    B. Degenerates
    C. Becomes considerably narrowed
    D. Becomes considerably widened

37. **Remnants of the dental lamina:**
    A. Do not persist throughout life
    B. Decrease in number but persist throughout life
    C. Remain constant in number with age
    D. Increase in number with age

38. **After dentin and enamel formation have reached the cementoenamel junction, the cervical loop:**
    A. Degenerates and disappears
    B. Forms the cell-free zone
    C. Forms the membrana preformativa
    D. Becomes transformed into the epithelial sheath of Hertwig

39. **When the continuity of Hertwig's sheath is destroyed following the beginning of dentin formation the result is?**
    A. Formation of epithelial rests of Malassez
    B. Formation of cementoblasts
    C. Development of epithelial diaphragm
    D. Differentiation of odontoblasts

40. **Odontoblasts:**
    A. Form the lateral foramina of the pulp
    B. Differentiate only where Hertwig's sheath is present
    C. Form interglobular dentin
    D. Can differentiate in the absence of Hertwig's sheath

41. **In three-rooted teeth:**
    A. The diaphragm surrounds three cervical openings
    B. Four epithelial fingers grow and fuse
    C. Three epithelial fingers grow and fuse and the diaphragm surrounds three cervical openings
    D. The diaphragm surrounds four cervical openings

42. **In developing tooth during formation of enamel and primary dentin:**
    A. The enamel is formed faster than the dentin
    B. The enamel is formed slower than the dentin
    C. The enamel is formed more cervically than the dentin
    D. The ameloblasts and odontoblasts move toward the pulp

43. **The shape of the root is determined by cells from the:**
    A. Dental papilla
    B. Dental organ
    B. Dental sac
    C. Vestibular lamina

44. **Hertwing's epithelial root sheath induces the formation of:**
    A. Enamel
    B. Coronal dentin
    C. Odontoblasts
    D. Ameloblasts

45. **During sixth week of embryonic life development of which structure is seen:**
    A. Hard palate   B. Soft palate
    C. Tooth   D. Oral epithelium

46. The formation of the Hertwig's epithelial root sheath occurs by:
    A. Dental lamina
    B. Enamel organ
    C. Stellate reticulum
    D. None of the above

47. The Hertwig's epithelial root sheath helps to:
    A. Form crown of tooth
    B. Form outer and inner enamel epithelium
    C. Mould the shape of roots
    D. All of the above

48. The droplets of enamel found in area of furcation of the roots of permanent molars are:
    A. Enamel organ
    B. Enamel cracks
    C. Enamel pearls
    D. Enamel spindle

ANSWERS

1. **D.** Dental lamina develops 2 or 3 weeks after the rupture of the buccopharyngeal membrane, which is a band of epithelium.

2. **D.** The distal proliferation of the dental lamina is responsible for the location of the germs of the permanent molars in the ramus of the mandible and the tuberosity of the maxilla.

3. **A.** The lingual extension of the dental lamina (suceessional lamina) develops from the fifth month *in utero* (permanent central incisor) to the tenth month of age (second premolar).

4. **C.** Refer to answer No. 3.

5. **A.** Refer to answer No. 3.

6. **C.** Remnants of the dental lamina persist as epithelial pearls or islands within the jaw as well as in the gingiva.

7. **A.** Refer to answer No. 6.

8. **D.** Vestibular lamina (lip furrow band) forms the oral vestibule.

9. **C.** The ectomesenchyme (neural crest cells) condenses to form dental papilla.

10. **D.** The primitive dental sac is formed by ectomesenchyme surrounding the enamel organ and dental papilla.

11. **A.** In the bad stage, the enamel organ consists of peripherally located low columnar cells and centrally located polygonal cells.

12. **D.** Enamel knot and enamel cord both are temporary structures that disappear before enamel formation begins.

13. **A.** Ameloblasts are tall columnar cells.

14. **B.** Membrana performativa represents the future dentino-enamel junction.

15. A. Hertwig's epithelial root sheath consists of the outer and inner enamel epithelia only.

16. C. Rests of Malassez have potential to form cysts.

17. B. Enamel pearls are sometimes found in the area of furcation of the roots of permanent molars.

18. A. If the continuity of Hertwig is root sheath is broken or is not established prior to dentine formation.

19. D. Abnormal initiation may result in the development of single or multiple supernumerary teeth.

20. D. Dentine formation therefore precedes and is essential to enamel formation. The differentiation of the epithelial cells precedes and is essential to the differentiation of the odontoblasts and the initiation of dentine formation. In vitamin A deficiency osteodentine is formed.

21. A. Hypopituitarism and hypothyroidism also result in small clinical crown that is often mistaken for a small anatomic crown.

22. C. The basic form and relative size of the future tooth, is established by morpho differentiation, that is, by differential growth.

23. A. Refer to answer No. 19

24. B. The dental papilla shows active budding of capillaries and mitotic figures, and its periphral cells adjacent to the inner enamel epithelium differentiate into the odontoblasts.

25. D. The lingual extension of dental lamina is called suceessional lamina.

26. A. Suceessional lamina is responsible for the development of permanent incisors, canines and premolars.

27. C. Permanent molars develop from a distal extension of the dental lamina.

28. B. After functional activity, the remnants of the dental lamina may persist in the gingiva or jaw in the form of islands or epithelial pearls.

29. **C.** These are developmental stages of tooth.

30. **D.** Histodifferentiation occurs in early bell stage white morphodifferentiation occurs in advanced bell stage.

31. **D.** After continuous division and differentiation in the cap stage, the size and shape of the enamel organ changes from knob-like to cap-like.

32. **C.** This proteinaceous fluid-containing albumin gives a cushion-like consistency to the stellate reticulum that supports and protects the delicate enamel forming cells.

33. **A.** All these structures are temporary and disappear before the beginning of amelogenesis. Probably their function is to act as a reservoir of dividing cells for the growing enamel organ.

34. **B.** Inner enamel epithelium consists of a single layer of tall columnar cells.

35. **C.** Stratum intermedium is essential for the development of enamel because it contains new ameloblasts and is essential for the formation and calcification of enamel.

36. **C.** When first few layers of dentine are laid down, the thickness of the stellate reticulum is reduced to facilitate the supply of nutritional elements to the formative cells.

37. **B.** After initiation of tooth development, the dental lamina degenerates.

38. **D.** Hertwig's epithelial root sheath contains only the outer and inner enamel epithelia.

39. **A.** These are found in the periodontal ligaments of the erupted teeth.

40. **B.** Enamel does not form in the absence of dentine. Dentine formation therefore precedes and is essential to enamel formation. The differentiation of epithelial cells precedes and is essential to the differentiation of the odontoblasts and the initiation of dentine formation.

41. **C.** If the continuity of Hertwig's root sheath is broken or is not established prior to dentine formation, a defect in the dentinal wall of the pulp ensues. This accounts for the development of accessory root canals opening on the periodontal surface of the root.

42. **B.** With the formation of dentine, the cells of the inner enamel epithelium differentiate into ameloblasts and enamel matrix is formed apposite the dentine. Enamel does not form in the absence of dentine.

43. **B.** The enamel organ (dental organ) forms Hertwig's epithelial root sheath, which molds the shape of the roots and initiates radicular dentine formation.

44. **C.** The cells of the inner layer of Hertwig's epithelial root sheath remain short and induce the differentiation of radicular cells into odontoblasts.

45. **C.** Dental lamina is formed during the 6th week of embroyonic life which serves as the primondium for the ectodermal portion of the deciduous teeth.

46. **B.** Hertwig's root sheath consists of the outer and inner enamel epithelia only and therefore it does not include the stratum intermedium and stellate retriculum.

47. **C.** Hertwig's root sheath also initiate radicular dentine formation.

48. **C.** If cells of the epithelial root sheath remain adherent to the dentine surface, they may differentiate into fully functioning ameloblasts and produce enamel. Such droplets of enamel, called enamel pearls, are sometimes found in the area of furcation of the roots of permanent molars.

Enamel

1. On the cusps of human molars and premolars, maximum thickness of enamel is about:
   A. 0 to 1 mm
   B. 2 to 3 mm
   C. 4 to 5 mm
   D. 4 to 6 mm

2. The specific gravity of enamel is:
   A. 2.4   B. 2.6
   C. 2.8   D. 3.0

3. Which of the following statement(s) is/are *true*?
   A. Enamel acts like a semipermeable membrane
   B. Enamel mainly consists of inorganic material (96%) and small amount of organic substance and water (4%)
   C. During development histologic staining reactions of enamel matrix resemble keratinizing epidermis
   D. All of the above

4. Which of the following statement(s) is/are *true*?
   A. Enamel is composed of enamel rods, rod sheath and interprismatic substances
   B. The number of enamel rods is about 5 million in lower lateral incisors and 12 million in the upper first molar
   C. The length of enamel rods is greater than thickness of enamel because of oblique direction and wavy course of the rods
   D. All of the above

5. The diameter of the enamel rods increases from dentino-enamel junction towards the surface of enamel in a ratio of about:
   A. 1:2   B. 1:3
   C. 1:4   D. 1:5

6. In cross sections of human enamel, many rods resemble:
   A. Triangle
   B. Fish scales
   C. Skin scales
   D. Cow horn

7. Which of the following statement(s) is/are *false*?
   A. The average thickness of the crystal of human enamel is about 30 nanometers
   B. The average width of the crystal of human enamel is about 90 namometer
   C. Both of the above
   D. None of the above

8. The striations are more pronounced in enamel that is:
   A. Sufficiently calcified
   B. Insufficiently calcified
   C. Fully calcified
   D. Not at all calcified

9. The enamel rods are segmented because the enamel matrix is formed in rhythmic manner. In humans these segments seem to be of a uniform length of about:
   A. 2 microns
   B. 4 microns
   C. 6 microns
   D. 8 microns

10. The arrangement of enamel rods in the permanent teeth, in the cervical region, deviates from the horizontal in an:
    A. Apical direction
    B. Occlusal direction
    C. Incisal direction
    D. All of the above

11. In an oblique plane the bundles of rods seem to intertwine more irregularly in the region of cusps or incisal edge, this optical appearance of enamel is called:
    A. Gnarled enamel
    B. Striation
    C. Hunter-Schreger bands
    D. Incremental lines of Retzius

12. The change in the direction of enamel rods is responsible for appearance of the:
    A. Gnarled enamel
    B. Hunter-Schreger bands
    C. Both of the above
    D. None of the above

13. The brownish bands i.e., the successive apposition of layer of enamel during the formation of crown is known as:
    A. Gnarled enamel
    B. Incremental line of Retzius
    C. Hunter-Schreger bands
    D. All of the above

14. In transverse sections of a tooth, the incremental line of Retzius appears as:
    A. Concentric circle
    B. Oblique line
    C. Zigzag line
    D. Cracks

15. Perikymata are transverse, wave-like grooves, believed to be the external manifestation of the:
    A. Striae of Retzius
    B. Gnarled enamel
    C. Hunter-Schreger bands
    D. All of the above

16. Perikymata are absent in the:
    A. Postnatal cervical part
    B. All permanent teeth
    C. All deciduous teeth
    D. Occlusal part of the deciduous teeth

17. The enamel of deciduous teeth develops partly before and partly after birth, the boundary between the two portions is known as:
    A. Basal lamina
    B. Incremental line
    C. Neonatal line
    D. Postnatal line

18. A delicate membrane which covers the entire crown of the newly erupted tooth is called as:
    A. Primary enamel cuticle
    B. Nasmyth's membrane
    C. Pellicle
    D. Both (A) and (B)

19. Thin, leaf-like structures that extend from enamel surface towards the dentino-enamel junction are called:
    A. Enamel tufts
    B. Gnarled enamel
    C. Enamel lamellae
    D. Enamel spindle

20. Which of the following statement(s) is/are *true* about enamel lamellae?
    A. Type A lamellae are composed of poorly calcified rod segments
    B. Type B lamellae consist of degenerated cells
    C. Type C lamellae arise in erupted teeth where cracks are filled with organic matter (more common)
    D. All of the above

21. Enamel tufts which arise at the dentinoenamel junction and reach into enamel to about 1/5th to 1/3rd of its thickness are:
    A. Hypocalcified enamel rods and interprismatic substances
    B. Hypercalcified enamel rods only
    C. Hypomineralized enamel rods only
    D. Similar to surface structures

22. In the mature dental tissues, the only tissue whose cells are lost is:
    A. Dentin   B. Pulp
    C. Cementum   D. Enamel

23. Which statement about enamel prism rod is *not correct*?
    A. The prisms run from the dentinoenamel junction to the crown surface
    B. The maximal width of a prism in horizontal section is 5 mm
    C. Prisms are wider near the dentinoenamel junction than near the crown surface
    D. The lengths of all enamel prisms are equal

24. **The enamel organ:**
    A. Promotes the differentiation of the dental papilla
    B. Does not form the enamel
    C. Does not narrow after the first layer of dentin has formed
    D. Does not promote the differentiation of the dentin

25. **After the enamel is completely formed and has undergone maturation:**
    A. The ameloblasts form the primary enamel cuticle
    B. The ameloblasts become much longer
    C. The enamel organ becomes a widened layer of stratified squamous epithelium
    D. None of the above

26. **During enamel maturation:**
    A. Calcification ceases
    B. Additional calcification occurs until complete calcification is present
    C. The ameloblasts play no role
    D. Additional enamel matrix is produced

27 . **The maturation of the enamel starts at:**
    A. Any point between occlusal surface and cervical region
    B. Occlusal surface of the crown and progresses toward cervical region
    C. Cervical region of the crown
    D. None of the above

28. **The formation of dentin:**
    A. Decreases the blood supply
    B. Is not based on tissue interdependence
    C. Is apparently a necessary stimulus for the formation of enamel
    D. Is not a necessary stimulus for the formation of enamel

29. **The perikymata are:**
    A. Elevations between the imbrication lines of Pickerill
    B. Present in the cementum
    C. Present in the enamel
    D. Present in the dentin

30. **The incremental lines of Retzius are seen in ground transverse sections:**
    A. As white bands not in concentric rings
    B. As brown bands not in concentric rings
    C. As concentric circles in the enamel which resemble rings in a tree trunk
    D. Running inward from the dentinoenamel junction

31. **The enamel rod sheath:**
    A. Has cross striations
    B. Has a lesser amount of inorganic matter than the enamel rod
    C. Is a more calcified enamel peripheral shell around each enamel rod
    D. None of the above

32. **The enamel rods in the incisal and cuspal areas are:**
    A. Vertical in direction
    B. Horizontal in direction
    C. Inclined apically
    D. Oblique and then horizontal in direction

33. **Enamel rods:**
    A. Have only a concave surface in cross section
    B. Increase in thickness from the dentinoenamel junction to the surface of enamel
    C. Are always the same thickness regardless of location
    D. Decrease in thickness from the dentinoenamel junction to the enamel surface

34. **Gnarled enamel is:**
    A. Present only at the cementoenamel junction
    B. Present only at the dentinoenamel junction
    C. Present only in deciduous teeth
    D. Due to markedly wavy and irregular enamel rods at the cusps or incisal edges

35. **Ionic interchanges between matured/erupted enamel and saliva:**
    A. Occur throughout life
    B. Occur only for two years following eruption
    C. Cease to occur in young adult life
    D. Do not occur

36. **Matured enamel is subjected to:**
    A. Erosion and attrition only
    B. Caries, erosion and attrition
    C. Caries and attrition only
    D. Caries and erosion only

37. **Enamel contains:**
    A. 96% organic substance
    B. 1.5% inorganic substance
    C. 100% organic substance
    D. None of the above

38. **Enamel contains:**
    A. 96% water
    B. 1% water
    C. 5% water
    D. None of the above

39. **Enamel is:**
    A. The only tissue whose formation does not cease
    B. Made up of 100% inorganic material
    C. The only calcified tissue in mammals of epithelial origin
    D. None of the above

40. **Enamel lamellae:**
    A. Are club-like swellings extending into the enamel for short distance
    B. Extend for short distances from the dentinoenamel junction toward the enamel surface
    C. Represent a pathway for proteolytic bacteria to the dentinoenamel junction
    D. Contain less organic matter than the enamel proper

41. **Enamel tufts:**
    A. Form a pathway for proteolytic bacteria to extend to the dentinoenamel junction
    B. Contain less organic material than normal enamel
    C. Contain highly calcified enamel rods and interprismatic substance
    D. Are areas of imperfect calcification extending for short distances from the dentinoenamel junction toward the enamel surface

42. **The Hunter-Schreger bands are:**
    A. Not visible in ground sections
    B. An illusion in reflected light
    C. Due to alternating directions of successive groups of enamel rods in reflected light
    D. Not visible in reflected light

43. **The uptake of fluorine by enamel:**
    A. Fails to taper off
    B. Is the same during the first years following enamel formation and in later years
    C. Is very slow during the first years following enamel formation
    D. Is very rapid during the first years following enamel formation

44. **Nitrogen is present in the surface enamel in:**
    A. Greater concentration in young teeth
    B. Greater concentration in older teeth
    C. Lower concentration in older teeth
    D. Lower concentration at the dentinoenamel junction

45. **The addition of 1 PPM of fluorine (F) to the drinking water causes:**
    A. An increment of about 300 PPM in surface enamel
    B. A decrement of about 100 PPM in surface enamel
    C. An increase in aluminum in the surface enamel
    D. No change in F concentration in surface enamel

46. **The principal blood supply of ameloblasts during most of enamel formation is from:**
    A. Enamel
    B. Dental pulp
    C. Reduced dental organ
    D. Dentin

47. **In cross section enamel prisms approximately have an average thickness of:**
    A. 3 microns
    B. 300 angstroms
    C. 3 angstroms
    D. 30 microns

48. **The long axis of enamel crystals is:**
    A. Parallel to the prism axis
    B. Parallel to the tooth surface
    C. Perpendicular to the tooth surface
    D. Both (A) and (C)

49. **The gnarled enamel is observed in:**
    A. In cervical area
    B. Only in the canines
    C. In carious areas
    D. In cuspal areas

50. **The enamel spindle is:**
    A. part of Tomes' enamel process
    B. The distal part of an odontoblastic process in enamel
    C. An area with a high collagen content
    D. A hypercalcified area

51. **Hunter-Schreger bands appear due to:**
    A. Daily growth rhythms
    B. Increased organic content in some areas
    C. Dietary change after birth
    D. Changes in the enamel prism orientation from one group of prisms to the next group of prisms

52. **Tomes' enamel process:**
    A. Remains in the mature enamel as the ameloblastic process
    B. Extends into the dentin
    C. Forms at the proximal end of the ameloblast
    D. Is apical to the terminal bar/area at the secretory apical end of ameloblast

53. **Enamel that can withstand severe masticatory force is:**
    A. Root enamel
    B. Cervical enamel
    C. Gnarled enamel
    D. Enamel lamellae

54. **Poorly calcified enamel is present in:**
    A. Perikymata   B. Gnarled enamel
    C. Enamel lamellae   D. Enamel prisms

55. **In the human body the hardest calcified tissue is:**
    A. Dentin
    B. Cementum
    C. Bone
    D. Enamel

56. **The percentage of the inorganic component of the enamel is:**
    A. 96%
    B. 95%
    C. 92%
    D. 90%

57. **The dentinoenamel junction is in the form of:**
    A. A scalloped line with convexities towards the enamel
    B. A scalloped line with the convexities of the scallops towards dentin
    C. A straight line
    D. None of the above

58. **Direction of the enamel rods in the deciduous and permanent teeth is:**
    A. Same throughout
    B. Different at cervical third
    C. Different at occlusal and incisal thirds
    D. None of the above

59. **For the control of dental caries fluoride level in drinking water should be:**
    A. 8 PPM
    B. 4 PPM
    C. 2 PPM
    D. 1 PPM

60. **Enamel tufts:**
    A. Arise from the surface of enamel and reach at dentinoenamel junction
    B. Arise at the dentinoenamel junction and proceed into the enamel towards surface
    C. Arise at dentin pulp junction and reach up to enamel
    D. Arise from the surface of enamel and reach up to the pulp

ANSWERS

1. **B.** On the cusps of human molars and premolars the enamel attains maximum thickness of 2 to 2.5 mm, thinning down to almost a knife edge of the neck of the tooth.

2. **C.** Enamel can act like a semipermeable membrane.

3. **D.** Chemical analysis of the matrix of mature enamel indicate that the amino acid composition is related to keratin and is distinctly different from collagen.

4. **D.** The rods located in the cusps, the thickest part of the enamel are longer than those of the cervical areas of the teeth.

5. **A.** The diameter of the enamel rods averages 4 µm.

6. **B.** In cross section under the light microscope enamel rods occasionally appear hexagonal.

7. **D.** The average width of the crystal of human enamel is three times than the thickness.

8. **B.** The enamel rods are segmented because the enamel matrix is formed in a rhythmic manner.

9. **B.** Enamel rod is built up of segments separated by dark lines that give it a striated appearance.

10. **A.** In the cervical and central part of the crown of a deciduous tooth, enamel rods are approximately horizontal.

11. **A.** Enamel rods are almost vertical in the region of the edge or tip of the cusps.

12. **C.** narled enamel is seen especially near the dentine in the region of the cusps or incisal edges.   unter   chreger bands can best be seen in a longitudinal ground section under obli ue reflected light.

13. **B.** They may be compared to the growth rings in the cross section of a tree.

14. **A.** In ground section, they appear as brownish bands. In longitudinal sections, they surround the tip of the dentine.

15. **A.** Perikymata are continuous around a tooth and usually lie parallel to each other and to the cementoenamel junction.

16. **D.** There are about 30 perikymata per millimeter in the region of the cementoenamel junction and their concentration gradually decreases to about 10 per millimeter near the occlusal or incisal edge of the surface.

17. **C.** Neonatal line or neonatal ring is an accentuated incremental line of Retzius.

18. **D.** This membrane is apparently secreted by the ameloblasts when enamel formation is completed.

19. **C.** Enamel lamellae consist of organic material, with but little mineral content. They may develop in planes of tension.

20. **D.** Lamellae of type A are restricted to the enamel, those of type B and C may reach into the dentine.

21. **A.** Tufts extend in the direction of the long axis of the crown therefore they are seen abundantly in horizontal sections.

22. **D.** When the enamel has completely developed and has fully calcified, the cell layers of stratum intermedium, outer enamel epithelium and ameloblasts form a stratified epithelial covering of the enamel, the so called reduced enamel epithelium.

23. **D.** They are estimated to vary between 0.05 and 1 μm.

24. **A.** It appears that the presence of dentine is necessary for the beginning of enamel matrix formation just as it was necessary for the epithelial cells to come in close proximity with the connective tissue of the pulp during differention of the odontoblasts and the beginning of dentine formation.

25. **A.** Maturation starts before the matrix has reached its full thickness.

26. **B.** The rod maturation takes place from dentine side and the sequence of rod maturation is from cusp tips and incisal edges of the crown towards the cervical line.

27. **B.** Under the organising influence of the proliferating epithelium of the enamel organ, the ectomesenchyme (neural crest cells) proliferates to form the dental papilla.

28. **C.** Primary enamel cuticle covers the enfore a crown of the newly erupted tooth but is probably soon removed by mastication. This membrane is a typical basal lamina apparently secreted by the ameloblasts when enamel formation is completed.

29. **C.** Perikymata are external manifestations of the striae of Retzius.

30. **C.** They appear as brownish bands in ground sections of the enamel.

31. **B.** Enamel rod sheath is more acid resistant than the enamel rod.

32. **A.** The rods are oriented at right angles to the dentine surface.

33. **B.** Diameter of the enamel rods increases from the dentino-enamel junction toward the surface of the enamel at a ratio of about 1:2.

34. **D.** In an oblique plane especially near the dentine in the region of cusps or incisal edges the bundles of the rods seem to intertwine more irregularly. This optical appearance of the enamel is called gnarled enamel.

35. **A.** Localized increase of certain elements such as nitrogen and fluorine, have been found in the superficial enamel layers of older teeth.

36. **B.** The most apparent age change in enamel is attrition or wear of the occlusal surfaces and proximal contact points as a result of mastication.

37. **D.** Enamel consists mainly of inorganic material (96%) and only a small amount of organic substance and water (4%).

38. **D.** Refer to answer No. 37.

39. **C.** When the enamel has completely developed and has fully calcified, the ameloblasts cease to be arranged in a well-defined layer and can no longer be differentiated from

the cells of the stratum intermedium and outer enamel epithelium.

40. **C.** Enamel lamellae may develop in planes of tension. Where rods cross such a plane, a short segment of the rod may not fully calcify.

41. **D.** Enamel tufts are seen abundantly in horizontal and rarely in longitudinal sections.

42. **C.** Hunter-Schreger bands can best be seen in a longitudinal ground section under oblique reflected light.

43. **D.** Where the drinking water contains fluoride in excess of 1.5 PPM, chronic endemic fluorosis may occur as a result of continuous use throughout the period of amelogenesis.

44. **B.** This suggests a continuous uptake by the enamel, probably from oral environment during aging.

45. **A.** The most effective means for mass control of dental caries has been adjustment of the fluoride level in communal water supplies to 1ppm.

46. **C.** The first appearance of dentine seems to be a critical phase in the life cycle of the inner enamel epithelium. As long as it is in contact with the connective tissue of the dental papilla, it receives nutrient material from the blood vessels of this tissue. When dentine forms, however, it cuts off the ameloblasts from their original source of nourishment, and from then they are supplied by the capillaries that surround and may even penetrate the outer enamel epithelium. This reversal of nutritional source is characterized by proliferation of capillaries of the dental sac and by reduction and gradual disappearance of the stellate reticulum.

47. **B.** When cut in cross-section, the crystals of human enamel are somewhat irregular in shape and have an average thickness of about 30 nm (300A degree) and an average width of about 90 μm (900 A degree)

48. **D.** Studies with polarized light and X-ray diffraction have indicated that the appatite crystals are arranged

approximately parallel to the long axis of the prisms. Electron microscopy revealed that they are approximately parallel to the long axes of the rods in their bodies or heads and deviate by about 65 degree from this axis as they fan out into the tails of the prisms.

49. **D.** The bundles of enamel rods seems to intertwine more irregularly giving rise the optical appearance of gnarled enamel.

50. **B.** Enamel spindles seem to originate from processes of the odontoblasts that extended into the enamel epithelium before hard substances were formed.

51. **D.** Hunter-Schreger bands are functional adaptation, minimizing the risk of cleavage in the axial direction under the influence of occlusal masticatory forces.

52. **D.** Projections of the ameloblasts into the enamel matrix have been named Tomes' processes.

53. **C.** Gnarled enamel aids in resisting the high masticatory loads without fracture that the cusps have to bear.

54. **C.** Enamel lamellae consist of organic material, with little mineral content.

55. **D.** Because of its high content of mineral salts and their crystalline arrangement.

56. **A.** The inorganic material of the enamel is similar to apatite.

57. **B.** Dentinoenamel junction is about 30 μm thick.

58. **B.** In the cervical and central parts of the crown of a deciduous tooth, the enamel rods are approximately horizontal. In the cervical region of the crown of permanent tooth, the enamel rods deviate from the horizontal in an apical direction.

59. **D.** Small amount of fluoride (about 1 to 1.2 PPM) reduces susceptibility to dental caries without causing mottling.

60. **B.** Enamel tufts reach into the enamel to about one fifth to one third of its thickness.

Dentin

1. **Which of the following statement(s) is/are *true* about Dentinoenamel Junction (DEJ)?**
   A. The surface of dentin at the DEJ is pitted
   B. This relation assumes the firm hold of the enamel cap on dentine surface
   C. DEJ appears as a scalloped line
   D. All of the above

2. **Which of the following statement(s) is/are *true* about Dentinoenamel Junction (DEJ)? DEJ is observed a:**
   A. Hypermineralized zone about 30 microns thick"
   B. Hypomineralized zone about 30 microns thick"
   C. Hypermineralized zone about 60 microns thick"
   D. Hypomineralized zone about 60 microns thick"

3. **Odontoblastic process which passes across the dentino-enamel junction into enamel is called:**
   A. Gnarled enamel
   B. Enamel spindle
   C. Enamel lamellae
   D. Enamel tufts

4. **Enamel spindle in ground section of dried teeth appears dark in:**
   A. Transmitted light
   B. Reflected light
   C. Polarized light
   D. All of the above

5. **In ground section of dried teeth, which of the following appear light in transmitted light?**
   A. Enamel spindle
   B. Dead tracts
   C. Sclerotic dentin
   D. All of the above

6. Dental lamellae may also be predisposing locations for caries because they contain:
   A. Much organic material
   B. Less organic material
   C. Much inorganic material
   D. None of the above

7. At the free border of the enamel organ, the outer and inner enamel epithelial layers are continuous and are reflected into one another as the:
   A. Facial loop
   B. Buccal loop
   C. Cervical loop
   D. Terminal bar

8. Which of the following statement(s) is/are *true*?
   A. Distal ends of enamel rods are not in direct contact with the dentin
   B. The projection of the ameloblasts into enamel matrix has been named Tomes' process
   C. Tomes' process contains rough endoplasmic reticulum and mitochondria
   D. All of the above

9. Which of the following statement(s) is/are *false*?
   A. At least two ameloblasts are involved in the synthesis of each enamel rod
   B. The bulk of the 'head' of each enamel rod is formed by one ameloblast while the contribution of 3 ameloblasts is to the component of the tail of each rod.
   C. Each ameloblast contributes to four different rods
   D. None of the above

10. The dentine is formed:
    A. Slightly before the enamel
    B. Slightly after the enamel
    C. Slightly after the cementum
    D. Slightly after periodontal ligament

11. Physically and chemically the dentine closely resembles:
    A. Enamel   B. Cementum
    C. Bone   D. Amalgam

12. The formula of hydroxyapatite is/are:
    A. $3 Ca_3 (PO_4)_2 Ca(OH)_2$
    B. $[Ca_{10}(OH)_2(PO_4)_6]$
    C. $CaSO_4 . 2H_2O$
    D. Both (A) and (B)

13. Hydroxyapatite crystal of dentine is:
    A. Much smaller than enamel
    B. Much larger than enamel
    C. Same as enamel
    D. None of the above

14. The ratio between outer and inner surfaces of dentine is about:
    A. 1:1
    B. 1:2
    C. 2:1
    D. 5:1

15. The ratio between the number of tubules per unit area on the pulpal and outer surfaces of dentine is about:
    A. 1:1   B. 1:2
    C. 4:1   D. 1:4

16. The main body of dentin is:
    A. Peritubular dentin
    B. Intertubular dentin
    C. Predentin
    D. Tomes' fibers

17. The first formed dentin which *is NOT* mineralized is:
    A. Peritubular
    B. Intertubular
    C. Predentin
    D. Odontoblastic process

18. The dentin that immediately surrounds the dentinal tubules is:
    A. Peritubular dentin
    B. Intertubular dentin
    C. Predentin
    D. First formed dentin

19. The cytoplasmic extension of the odontoblast into dentinal tubules is called as:
   A. Odontoblastic process
   B. Tomes' fibers
   C. None of the above
   D. Both (A) and (B)

20. The odontoblastic processes are composed of:
   A. Microtubules 20 microns in diameter
   B. Small filaments 5 to 7.5 microns in diameter
   C. Mitochondria
   D. All of the above

21. Secondary dentin is:
   A. First formed dentin
   B. Dentin formed before root completion
   C. Dentin formed after root completion
   D. Circumpulpal dentin

22. The incremental lines of Von Ebner are in:
   A. Enamel
   B. Dentin
   C. Bone
   D. Cementum

23. Some of the incremental lines are accentuated because of disturbances in the matrix and mineralization process and are known as Contour lines (Owen), and are found in :
   A. Enamel   B. Dentin
   C. Bone   D. Cementum

24. Contour lines (Owen) are:
   A. Hypocalcified bands
   B. Hypercalcified bands
   C. Non-mineralized bands
   D. None of the above

25. Sometimes mineralization of dentin begins in globular area; these hypomineralized zones are known as:
   A. Interglobular dentin
   B. Granular layer
   C. Peritubular dentin
   D. Intertubular dentin

26. Tomes' granular layer is caused by a coalescing and looping of the terminal portions of the dentinal tubules found in:
    A. Enamel
    B. Crown dentin
    C. Root dentin
    D. Cementum

27. Due to extensive abrasion, erosion, caries or operative procedures, the odontoblast deposits dentin which is called:
    A. Reparative dentin
    B. Secondary dentin
    C. Tertiary dentin
    D. Both (A) and (C) are correct

28. Dentin areas characterized by degenerated odontoblastic processes which appear white in reflected light are called as:
    A. Dead tracts
    B. Sclerotic dentin
    C. Transparent dentin
    D. Mantle dentin

29. Dead tracts are mostly found in:
    A. Only deciduous teeth
    B. Only incisors
    C. Older teeth
    D. Carious teeth

30. Which of the following statement(s) is/are *true* about sclerotic dentin?
    A. It leads to protective changes in the dentin itself
    B. The mineralization is very similar to peritubular dentin
    C. It appears dark in reflected light
    D. All of the above

31. How much initial increment of dentine is formed during dentinogenesis until the crown is formed?
    A. 3 μm/day
    B. 4 μm/day
    C. 5 μm/day
    D. 6 μm/day

32. **Korff's fibers are found in:**
    A. Primary dentin   B. Secondary dentin
    C. Sclerotic dentin   D. Transparent dentin

33. **What is the rate of reparative dentin formation after cavity preparation in dentin?**
    A. 4 microns per day
    B. 6 microns per day
    C. 8 microns per day
    D. 10 microns per day

34. **The apatite crystals of dentin are:**
    A. 300 times larger than those formed in enamel
    B. 300 times smaller than those formed in enamel
    C. 3000 times smaller than those formed in enamel
    D. 3000 times larger than those formed in enamel

35. **How many living cells are damaged when 1 mm^2 of dentin is exposed?**
    A. About 10,000 living cells
    B. About 20,000 living cells
    C. About 30,000 living cells
    D. About 40,000 living cells

36. **The rapid penetration and spread of caries in the dentin is the result of the:**
    A. Tubule system in the dentin
    B. Canaliculi system in the dentin
    C. Haversian system in the dentin
    D. All of the above

37. **The sulcular epithelium is:**
    A. Keratinized
    B. Nonkeratinized
    C. Orthokeratinized
    D. Parakeratinized

38. **The remnant of the primary enamel cuticle after eruption is referred to as:**
    A. Nasmyth's membrane
    B. Pellicle
    C. Primary attachment epithelium
    D. All of the above

39. The separation of primary attachment epithelium from the enamel is termed as:
   A. Active eruption
   B. Passive eruption
   C. Fast eruption
   D. Functional eruption

40. The clinical crown is the part of the tooth which is:
   A. Covered by enamel
   B. Covered by gingiva
   C. Exposed in the oral cavity
   D. None of the above

41. Compared with intertubular dentin, peritubular dentin is characterized by having:
   A. Less inorganic salt content and a heavier collagenous matrix
   B. More inorganic salt content and a finer collagenous matrix
   C. More fluid content and a different refractive index
   D. Fewer fibers and being more stainable

42. The most important property of clinical significance of dentin of the tooth is that it:
   A. Is softer than enamel
   B. Protects the pulp
   C. Supports the enamel
   D. Is more resilient than enamel

43. Growth in height of the alveolar process is dependant upon:
   A. Growth of alveolar process with the eruption of teeth.
   B. Condylar growth
   C. Growth of the upper face
   D. Growth of the cranial base

44. When teeth fail to develop in the jaw, the alveolar process:
   A. Shows partial growth
   B. Fails to form
   C. Continues to grow
   D. Shows excessive growth

45. The differentiation of odontoblasts and formation of dentin and enamel first begins at the:
   A. Region of the cervical loop
   B. Incisal edge or tip of cusps
   C. Midway between the incisal edge and cervical loop
   D. None of the above

46. **Growth centers in tooth development are located at:**
    A. Any region between the incisal edge and cervical loop
    B. The incisal edge and tip of the cusps
    C. The region of the cervical loop
    D. Dentinoenamel junction under the cusp tip

47. **In the formation of dentin:**
    A. Odontoblasts fail to recede towards the pulp
    B. Korff's fibers form the odontoblasts
    C. Korff's fibers are initially deposited dentin at the cusp tips
    D. Korff's fibers become homogenized and form predentin

48. **Predentin consists of:**
    A. Mineral salts and cementing substance
    B. Cementing substance
    C. Calcospherites
    D. None of the above

49. **When odontoblasts recede towards the pulp, they leave a part of their cytoplasm termed?**
    A. Korff's fibers
    B. Tomes' process within the formed dentin
    C. Membrana preformativa
    D. None of the above

50. **Dentin consists of:**
    A. Cells, collagen fibers and cementing substance
    B. Cementing substance
    C. Intercellular substances
    D. None of the above

51. **Which is highly calcified dentin?**
    A. Interglobular dentin
    B. Tomes' granular layer
    C. Peritubular dentin
    D. Intertubular dentin

52. **Dentin in which the tubules are calcified is termed as:**
    A. Physiological secondary dentin
    B. Dead tract dentin
    C. Interglobular dentin
    D. Sclerotic dentin

53. **Korff's fibers are:**
    A. The same as enamel spindles
    B. The same as the enamel tufts
    C. Related to reticular fibers
    D. Intracellular

54. **Important characteristic of mantle dentin is presence of:**
    A. Enamel spindles
    B. Hertwig's sheath
    C. Elastin fibers
    D. Korff's fibers

55. **Initially the neonatal line is:**
    A. Eliminated by fluoridated water
    B. Hypercalcified
    C. Found in all teeth
    D. Hypocalcified

56. **The percentage of the organic and inorganic components of dentin is:**
    A. 35% organic and water and 65% inorganic
    B. 35% inorganic and 65% organic and water
    C. 60% organic and water and 40% inorganic
    D. 50% organic and water and 50% inorganic

57. **The odontoblastic process is surrounded by the ring-shaped transparent zone called as:**
    A. Tubular dentin
    B. Peritubular dentin
    C. Intertubular dentin
    D. Ring dentin

58. **The diameters of the dentinal tubules are:**
    A. Smaller near the pulpal cavity
    B. Larger at their outer ends
    C. Larger near the pulp cavity
    D. Are same from pulp cavity to the outer ends

59. **The most peripheral part of the primary dentin is:**
    A. Intertubular dentin
    B. Predentin
    C. Mantle dentin
    D. Circumpulpal dentin

60. **Tertiary dentin is:**
    A. Reparative dentin
    B. Response dentin
    C. Reactive dentin
    D. All of the above

61. **When calcospherites fail to fuse during calcification of dentin matrix:**
    A. Transparent dentin is formed
    B. Irregular dentin is formed
    C. Interglobular dentin is formed
    D. Sclerotic dentin is formed

62. **Odontoblast cell bodies are present in the:**
    A. Enamel
    B. Dentin
    C. Pulp
    D. Cementum

ANSWERS

1. **D.** The convexities of the scallops of dentinoenamel junction are directed toward the dentin.

2. **A.** Dentinoenamel junction is most prominent before mineralization is complete.

3. **B.** They originate from odontoblastic processes that extended into the enamel epithelium before hard substances are formed. They are at right angle to the surface of dentin.

4. **A.** In ground section of dried teeth, the organic content of the spindles disintegrates and is replaced by air.

5. **C.** Transparent or sclerotic dentin can be observed in the teeth of elderly people, especially in the roots. It also appears dark in reflected light.

6. **A.** Enamel lamellae may be a site of weakness in a tooth and may form a road of entry for bacteria that initiate caries.

7. **C.** The inner and outer enamel epithelia are elsewhere separated from each other by a large mass of cells differentiated into two distinct layers-stratum intermedium and stellate reticulum.

8. **D.** The arrangement of Tomes' processes gives "Picket fence" appearance. Rods are at an angle to ameloblasts and Tomes's processes.

9. **D.** Each rod is formed by four ameloblasts.

10. **A.** The ameloblasts begin their secretary activity when a small amount of dentin has been laid down. The presence of dentin seems to be necessary for the beginning of enamel matrix formation.

11. **C.** The bone contains osteocytes, whereas the dentin contains only the processes of the cells that form it.

12. **D.** The inorganic component of dentin has been shown by X-ray diffraction to consist of hydroxyapatite, as in bone, cementum and enamel.

13. A. Hydroxyapatite crystals of dentin are plate shaped.

14. D. The dentinal tubules are more closely packed near the pulp.

15. C. Near the pulpal surface of dentin the number of dentinal tubules varys between 50,000 and 90,000 per square millimeter.

16. B. Although intertubular dentin is highly mineralized, the matrix, like bone and cementum is retained after decalcification.

17. C. The predentin is located adjacent to the pulp tissue, and is 2 to 6 μm wide.

18. A. Peritubular dentin is more highly mineralized (about 9%) than intertubular dentin.

19. D. These processes are largest in diameter near the pulp (3 to 4 μm) and taper to approximately 1μm further into the dentin.

20. D. The processes narrow to about half the size of the cell as they enter the tubules.

21. C. Secondary dentin contains fewer tubules than primary dentin.

22. B. They run at right angles to the dentinal tubules and reflect the daily rhythmic, recurrent deposition of dentin matrix.

23. B. Contour lines (owen) are readily demonstrated in ground sections. They represent hypocalcified bands.

24. A. Occasionally some of the incremental lines are accentuated because of the disturbances in the matrix and mineralization process called contour lines (owen) of dentin.

25. A. Interglobular dentin appears in crown dentin at short distance from the dentinoenamel junction. They appear black in transmitted light in ground section.

26. C. Tomes' granular layer is visualized in transmitted light.

27. **D.** Reparative dentin is characterized as having fewer and more twisted tubules than normal dentin. Sclerotic dentin appears transparent or light in transmitted light and dark in reflected light.

28. **A.** Dead tract areas demonstrate decreased sensitivity and appear to a greater extent in older teeth. They are probably the initial step in the formation of sclerotic dentin.

29. **C.** Refer to answer No. 28.

30. **D.** The tubule lumen is obliterated with mineral, which appears very much like the peritubular dentin.

31. **B.** After this time dentin production slows to about 1 μm/day.

32. **A.** Korff's fibers have been described as the initial dentin deposition along the cusp tips.

33. **A.** Dentinogenesis begins at the cusp tips after the odontoblasts have differentiated and begin collagen production.

34. **B.** The ultimate crystal size in dentin remains very small about 3 nm (30A degree) in thickness and 100nm (1000 A degree) in length.

35. **C.** It is advisable to seal the exposed dentin surface with a nonirritating, insulating substance.

36. **A.** The dentinal tubules form a passage for invading bacteria that may thus reach the pulp through a thick dentinal layer.

37. **B.** The sulcular epithelium lacks epithelial ridges.

38. **A.** When the ameloblasts finish formation of enamel matrix, they leave a thin membrane on the surface of enamel, the primary enamel cuticle.

39. **B.** Once the tip of the crown has emerged, the reduced enamel epithelium (primary enamel cuticle + epithelial enamel organ) is termed the primary attachment epithelium.

40. **C.** The part of tooth covered by enamel is anatomical crown.

41. B. Peritubular dentin is more highly mineralized (about 9%) than intertubular dentin.

42. D. Unlike enamel which is very hard and brittle, dentin is elastic and subject to slight deformation.

43. A. The alveolar process develops only during the eruption of teeth and it gradually diminishes in height after the loss of teeth.

44. A. Refer to answer No. 43.

45. B. Dentin formation begins of the late bell stage of development of tooth at the tip of the cusp. The root dentin forms later.

Differentiation into ameloblasts and production of enamel matrix first takes place in the regions of cusps and incisal edges and then proceeds toward the cervical loop.

46. D. Dentin and enamel formation begin at the late bell stage of development of tooth at the tip of the cusp. From here their formation spreads apically.

47. C. As each increment of predentin is formed along the pulpal border, it remains a day before it is calcified and the next increment of predentine forms.

48. D. It is first formed dentin and is not mineralized.

49. D. As the adontoblast recedes, it leaves behind a single extension, and the several initial processes join into one, which become enclosed in a tubule.

50. D. Dentin consists of 35% organic matter and water and 65% inorganic material. The organic substance consists of collagenous fibrils and a ground substance of muco-polysaccharides (proteoglycans and glycosaminogly-cans).

51. C. A very delicate organic matrix has been demonstrated in peritubular dentin that along with the mineral is lost after decalcification.

52. D. Causes of sclerotic or transparent dentin are caries, attrition, abrasion, erosion (wasting disease) and cavity preparation.

53. C. Korff's fibers are precollagenous or reticular or argyrophilic in nature.

54. D. Mantle dentin is the outer or most periphral part of the primary dentin and is about 20 µm thick.

55. D. It is an accentuated incremental line of Retzius in enamel or an accentuated contour line in dentin between prenatal and postnatal enamel or dentin respectively. It is seen in enamel and dentin of deciduous teeth and in the first permanent molars.

56. A. The inorganic component of dentin has been shown by X-ray diffraction to consists of hydroxyapatite as in bone, cementum and enamel.

57. B. Several investigators believe the calcified dentinal tubule has an inner organic lining termed the lamina limitans.

58. C. Diameter of dentinal tubules near the pulpal end is 3 to 4 µm and that at their outer end is 1µm.

59. C. It is the area of initial dentine matrix formation.

60. D. Reparative dentin is formed in response to extensive abrasion, erosion, caries or operative procedures after exposed or cut of the odontoblastic processes.

61. C. Interglobular dentin forms in the crowns of teeth in the circumpulpal dentin just below the mantle dentine and it follows the incremental pattern.

62. C. Odontoblastic processes are present in the dentinal tubules in dentin.

Dental Pulp

1. How many pulp organs are normally found in every person?
   A. 22
   B. 32
   C. 52
   D. 62

2. The total volume of all the permanent pulp organs is:
   A. 0.02 cc
   B. 0.006 cc
   C. 0.068 cc
   D. 0.38 cc

3. The total volume of pulp organ of maxillary first molar is:
   A. 0.006 cc
   B. 0.007 cc
   C. 0.068 cc
   D. 0.38 cc

4. The total volume of pulp organ of mandibular central incisor is:
   A. 0.006 cc
   B. 0.007 cc
   C. 0.012 cc
   D. 0.014 cc

5. The average diameter of the apical foramen of the mandibular and maxillary teeth in adults is:
   A. 0.3 mm and 0.4 respectively
   B. 0.6 mm and 0.7mm respectively
   C. 0.8 mm and 0.9 mm respectively
   D. 0.8 mm and 0.6 mm respectively

6. Weil's zone of pulp is a:
   A. Cell-rich zone
   B. Cell-free zone
   C. Fibroblast zone
   D. Mesenchymal cell zone

7. The most numerous cell type in the pulp is:
   A. Fibroblast
   B. Cementoblast
   C. Odontoblast
   D. Defense cell

8. In the young pulp the cells, which divide and are active in protein synthesis are known as:
   A. Fibroblasts
   B. Fibrocytes
   C. Odontoblasts
   D. Histiocytes

9. The primary cells in the very young pulp, which may become odontoblasts, fibroblasts or macrophages when needed, are:
   A. Undifferentiated mesenchyme cells
   B. Defense cells
   C. Plasma cells
   D. Rough endoplasmic reticulum

10. The anastomosis which occurs in pulp is:
    A. Venous-venous
    B. Arteriole-venous
    C. Both (A) and (B)
    D. None of the above

11. The second most prominent cell in the pulp is:
    A. Fibroblast   B. Odontoblast
    C. Cementoblast   D. Neutrophil

12. Lymph vessels draining the pulp and periodontal ligament of mandibular anterior teeth pass to the:
    A. Submental lymph nodes
    B. Submandibular lymph nodes
    C. Deep cervical lymph nodes
    D. All of the above

13. Sensation of pain in pulp is mediated by:
    A. Large myelinated fibers
    B. Large unmyelinated fibers
    C. Small unmyelinated fibers
    D. None of the above

14. The peripheral axons form a network of nerves located adjacent to the cell rich zone in pulp   known as:
    A. 5 HT
    B. Plexus of Rashkow
    C. Zone of Weil
    D. Brachial plexus

15. Sensory response in the pulp can differentiate between:
    A. Heat and pain
    B. Touch and heat
    C. Pressure and chemicals
    D. None of the above

16. Which of the following statement(s) is/are *true*?
    A. Pulpal pressure is among the highest of the body tissues
    B. Sensory nerves in the pulp respond with pain to all stimuli
    C. Function of pulp is inductive, formative, nutritive, protective and defensive
    D. All of the above

17. The average length of time a deciduous pulp functions in the oral cavity is only about:
    A. 8.3 years
    B. 10.3 years
    C. 11.3 years
    D. 13.3 years

18. The maximum life of the deciduous pulp including both prenatal and postnatal times of   development and the period of regression is approximately:
    A. 8.3 years
    B. 9.6 years
    C. 10.6 years
    D. 12.6 years

19. Which of the following statement(s) is/are *true* about regressive changes of pulp?
    A. Mitochondria and endoplasmic reticulum are reduced in number and size
    B. Fibrosis of pulp
    C. Pulp stones and diffuse calcifications of pulps
    D. All of the above

20. Calcification in the walls of blood vessels in aging pulp is found most often in the region near the:
    A. Coronal portion of root
    B. CEJ of root
    C. Apical foramen
    D. Pulp chamber

21. Calcification of thrombi in blood vessels is called:
    A. True denticle
    B. Diffuse calcification
    C. Phlebolith
    D. All of the above

22. The structures similar to dentin in that they exhibit dental tubuli containing the process of odontoblasts, are rarely found and located close to the apical foramen, are:
    A. True denticles
    B. False denticles
    C. Cementicles
    D. None of the above

23. Which of the following statement(s) is/are *true*?
    A. Diffuse calcifications are usually found in the root canal and less often in coronal pulp
    B. Denticles are seen more frequently in the coronal pulp
    C. 90% of teeth in persons over the age of 50 years contain calcification of some type
    D. All of the above

24. The tooth pulp is initially called the:
    A. Predentin
    B. Dental papilla
    C. Subpulpal dentin
    D. Pulp polyp

25. At the location of future incisor the development of the dental pulp begins at about:
    A. 4th week of embryonic life
    B. 6th week of embryonic life
    C. 8th week of embryonic life
    D. 9th week of embryonic life

26. The cell of the dental pulp that has the potential for giving rise to several distinctly different types of cells is the:
    A. Endothelial cell
    B. Mesenchymal cell
    C. Schwann cell
    D. Macrophage

27. After completion of root formation, the remainder of the dental papilla becomes the:
    A. Hertwig's sheath
    B. Dental pulp
    C. Dental follicle
    D. Enamel organ

28. The cells that line the pulp chambers of newly erupted teeth are:
    A. Ameloblasts
    B. Odontoblasts
    C. Fibroblasts
    D. Cementoblasts

29. The function of non-myelinated sympathetic nerve endings in the pulp is to:
    A. Form a plexus in the cell free zone of Weil
    B. Elicit only a pain response
    C. Alter the blood flow to the pulp
    D. Enter the dentinal tubules

30. The coronal pulp has:
    A. Two surfaces
    B. Four surfaces
    C. Five surfaces
    D. Six surfaces

31. The majority of the nerves that enter the pulp are:
    A. Myelinated
    B. Non-myelinated
    C. Both of the above
    D. None of the above

32. Dental pulp functions:
    A. To protect the tooth by its phagocytic cells
    B. As a source of odontoblasts
    C. To provide sensitivity to heat, cold and pressure.
    D. All of the above

33. **Wandering cells of pulp are:**
    A. Lymphoid wandering cells
    B. Histiocytes
    C. Fibroblasts
    D. Undifferentiated mesenchymal cells

34. **True denticles:**
    A. Have dental tubules and the processes of the odontoblasts
    B. Are usually located close to the apical foramen
    C. May be induced by fragments of epithelial root sheath
    D. All of the above

35. **Which of the following statement(s) is/are *true*?**
    A. The free denticles are entirely surrounded by pulp tissue
    B. Attached denticles are partly fused with the dentin
    C. Embedded denticles are entirely surrounded by dentin
    D. All are correct

36. **The incidence and size of pulp stone:**
    A. Decrease with age
    B. Increase with age
    C. There is no effect of age
    D. None of the above

37. **The vitality of the pulp depends upon:**
    A. Nerve supply
    B. Blood supply
    C. Both of the above
    D. None of the above

38. **When compared with a very young pulp, the more aged pulp contains?**
    A. Fewer cells and fewer collagen fibers
    B. More cells and fewer collagen fibers
    C. Fewer cells and more collagen fibers
    D. More cells and more collagen fibers

39. **Which cell type is usually *not found* in dental pulp?**
    A. Small lymphocytes and plasma cells
    B. Fat cells
    C. Histiocytes and macrophages
    D. Fibroblasts and undifferentiated mesenchymal cells

40. In an inflamed pulp usually there are certain cells which are associated with small blood vessels having large and prominent nucleus, these are:
    A. Lymphocytes
    B. Mast cells
    C. Histiocytes
    D. Fibroblasts

41. The blood flow in vessels of the pulp as compared to most of the other organs of the body is:
    A. Very slow
    B. Faster
    C. Almost nil
    D. Equal

42. The proof of presence of lymph capillaries in the pulp are on the basis of:
    A. Absence of basal lamina adjacent to the endothelium
    B. Absence of red blood cells and presence of lymphocytes in certain vessels
    C. Injected fine particulate substances subsequently found in some thin walled vessels other than blood vessels
    D. All of the above

43. Which of the following fibers are *not found* in dental pulp?
    A. Argyrophilic fibers
    B. Collagen fibers
    C. Elastic fibers
    D. None.

ANSWERS

1. **C.** After dentin production begins, the dental papilla is designated as the pulp organ. Each tooth has a pulp organ and total number of teeth in whole life span is fifty-two.

2. **D.** The mean volume of a single adult human pulp is 0.02 CC.

3. **C.** Permanent maxillary first molar has the maximum volume of pulp.

4. **A.** Permanent mandibular central incisor has the lowest volume of pulp.

5. **A.** The location and shape of the apical foramen may undergo changes as a result of functional influences on the teeth.

6. **B.** It is a space in which the odontoblasts may move pulpward during tooth development and later to a limited extent in functioning teeth.

7. **A.** Fibroblasts function in collagen fiber formation throughout the pulp during the life of the tooth.

8. **B.** In the older pulp fibrocytes appear rounded or spindle shaped with short processes and exhibit fewer intracellular organelles.

9. **A.** Undifferentiated mesenchymal cells are distinctive because they lack a ribosome-bounded endoplasmic reticulum and have mitochondria with readily discernible cisternae.

10. **C.** The arteriole-venous shunts may have an important role in regulation of pulpal blood flow.

11. **B.** The processes of the odontoblasts contain no endoplasmic reticulum.

12. **A.** Lymph vessels of pulp draining the posterior teeth pass to the submandibular and deep cervical lymph nodes.

13. **A.** The majority of the nerves that enter the pulp are non-myelinated.

14. **B.** It is also called as parietal layer of nerves.

15. **D.** This is because the pulp organs lack those types of receptors that specifically distinguish other stimuli.

16. **D.** The flow of blood in arterioles of pulp is 0.3 to 1 mm per second, in venules approximately 0.15 mm per second and in capillaries about 0.08 mm per second.

17. **A.** The maximum life of the primary pulp including both prenatal and postnatal times of development and the period of regression is 9.6 years.

18. **B.** Refer to answer No. 17.

19. **D.** Cells of pulp also decreases in size and number.

20. **C.** Diffuse calcifications are usually found in the root canal and less often in the coronal area, whereas denticles are seen more frequently in the coronal pulp.

21. **C.** Phleboliths may also serve as nidi for false denticles.

22. **A.** Development of true denticle is caused by the inclusion of remnants of the epithelial root sheath within the pulp.

23. **D.** True denticles are comparatively rare and are usually located close to the apical foramen.

24. **B.** The dental papilla is designated as pulp only after dentin forms around it.

25. **C.** The dental papilla controls early tooth formation. It also controls whether the forming enamel organ is to be an incisor or a molar.

26. **B.** Undifferentiated mesenchymal cells are the primary cells in the very young pulp. They are believed to be totipotent cells.

27. **B.** Dental papilla controls early tooth formation.

28. **B.** Odontoblaste are the second most prominent cells in the pulp.

29. **C.** The large myelinated fibers mediate the sensation of pain that may be caused by external stimuli.

30. **D.** The coronal pulp in young individuals resembles the shape of the outer surface of the crown dentin.

31. **B.**   The nonmyelinated nerves are found in close association with the blood vessels of the pulp and many are sympathetic in nature.

32. **D.**   Dental pulp functions as inductive, formative, nutritive, protective and defensive or reparative.

33. **B.**   The distinguishing feature of macrophages or histiocytes is aggregates of vesicles or phagosome which contain phagocytized dense irregular bodies.

34. **A.**   True denticles are comparatively rare and are usually located close to the apical foramen.

35. **D.**   All types of denticles are believed to be formed free in the pulp and later to become attached or embedded as dentin formation progresses.

36. **B.**   All pulp stones or denticles begin as small nodules but increase in size by incremental growth on their surface.

37. **B.**   Vitalometers provide information about the status of the nerves supplying the pulpal tissue and therefore, check the sensitivity of the pulp and not its vitality. The vitality of the pulp depends on its blood supply and one can have teeth with damaged nerve but normal blood supply (as in case of traumatized teeth). Such pulps do not respond to electrical or thermal stimuli but are completely viable in every respect.

38. **C.**   Hence the reparative capacity of the aged pulp is reduced.

39. **B.**   Fibroblasts are the most numerous cell types in the pulp.

40. **C.**   Histiocytes are defense cells. Their presence is disclosed by intravital dyes such as trypan blue.

41. **B.**   The pulpal pressure is among the highest of the body tissues.

42. **D.**   Lymph nodes, those of the posterior teeth pass to the submandibular and deep cervical lymph nodes.

43. **C.**   Collagen fibers in the pulp exhibit typical cross striations at 64 nm (640 Å) and range in length from 10 to 100 nm or more.

Cementum

1. **Cementum was first demonstrated microscopically in:**
   A. 1835
   B. 1935
   C. 1895
   D. 1995

2. **The cementum is:**
   A. Vascular
   B. Avascular
   C. Attached to pulp
   D. None of the above

3. **Which of the following statement(s) is/are *true*?**
   A. Young cementum is lighter in color than dentin
   B. Cementum is permeable
   C. Cementum has the highest fluoride content of all the mineralized tissues
   D. All of the above

4. **Epithelial rests of Malassez are found in the:**
   A. Dentin
   B. Periodontal ligament
   C. Cementum
   D. Enamel

5. **The uncalcified matrix of cementum is called:**
   A. Cementoid
   B. True denticles
   C. False denticles
   D. Free denticles

6. **Which of the following statement(s) is/are *true*?**
   A. Acellular cementum is often missing on the apical 3rd of the root
   B. Cementum is thinnest at the cemento-enamel junction
   C. Cementum is thickest at the apex
   D. All of the above

7. **The incremental lines of cementum are:**
   A. Poorly mineralized
   B. Highly mineralized
   C. Irregularly mineralized
   D. None of the above

8. **In approximately 60% of teeth:**
   A. Cementum overlaps the enamel at the cervical end for a short distance
   B. Cementum and enamel do not meet
   C. Cementum meets in a sharp line to enamel
   D. A connective tissue attachment to tooth is possible without cementum

9. **Absence of cementum is found in:**
   A. Hypophosphatasia
   B. Hyperparathyroidism
   C. Hyperthyroidism
   D. Mongolism

10. **Which of the following statement(s) is/are *true*?**
    A. Cementum is not resorbed under normal conditions
    B. Deposition of cementum in an apical area can compensate for loss of tooth substance by occlusal wear
    C. Hypercementosis is abnormal thickening of cementum
    D. All of the above

11. **Orthodontic tooth movement is made possible because:**
    A. Cementum is more resistant to resorption than bone
    B. Bone is more resistant to resorption than cementum
    C. Bone is poorly vascularized than cementum
    D. Cementum is poorly vascularized than bone

12. **Regarding functional repair of cementum which of the following statement(s) is/are *correct*?**
    A. There is tendency to reestablish the former outline of root surface
    B. Only a thin layer of cementum is deposited on the surface of deep resorption and root outline is not reconstructed
    C. The outline of alveolar bone in these cases follows that of root surface
    D. Both (B) and (C)

13. **Compact bone and cellular cementum are similar as they contain:**
    A. Canaliculi and incremental lines
    B. Lacunae and elastic fibers
    C. Collagen fibers and blood vessels
    D. Sharpey's fibers and elastic fibers

14. **Sharpey's fibers:**
    A. Arise from Hertwig's sheath
    B. Arise from the epithelial rests of Malassez
    C. Arise from the epithelial diaphragm
    D. Are collagen fibers of the dental follicle embedded in the cementum

15. **Cementoid is:**
    A. The alveolar bone
    B. The central zone of fibers
    C. The uncalcified cementum
    D. The calcified matrix of cementum

16. **Cementum formation is:**
    A. Not a continuous process
    B. Always results in cellular cementum
    C. A continuous process
    D. Present in the dental follicle

17. **Cementum is formed from:**
    A. Endoderm
    B. The dental organ
    C. Ectoderm
    D. The dental sac

18. **Cellular cementum is thickest:**
    A. Around the root apex
    B. At cementoenamel junction
    C. At middle one third of the root
    D. At coronal one third of the root

19. **Cementum is thinnest at:**
    A. Apical third of root
    B. Middle third of root
    C. Cementoenamel junction
    D. Apical foramen

20. **Acellular cementum is thickest at:**
    A. Apical foramen
    B. Coronal one third of root
    C. Middle one third of root
    D. Apical one third of root

21. **Cementum overlaps the cervical end of enamel in a relatively sharp line in:**
    A. 30% of teeth
    B. 20% of teeth
    C. 10% of teeth
    D. None

22. **If functional qualities of cementum improve by its overgrowth, it is called as:**
    A. Hypoplasia
    B. Hyperplasia
    C. Hypertrophy
    D. Any of the above

23. **In a nonfunctioning teeth there is:**
    A. Thickening of the cementum
    B. Thinning of the cementum
    C. No change in cementum
    D. None of the above

ANSWERS

1. **A.** It is a specialized connective tissue that shares some physical, chemical and structural characteristics with compact bone.

2. **B.** Cementum is somewhat lighter in color than dentin.

3. **D.** Under clinical conditions, it is not possible to distinguish cementum from dentin-based on color alone.

4. **B.** The formation of the periodontal ligaments occurs after the cells of Hertwig epithelial root sheath have separated, forming the strands known as the epithelial rests of Malassez.

5. **A.** Cementum contains 50% to 55% organic material and water.

6. **D.** Acellular cementum usually predominates in the cononal half of the root.

7. **B.** Incremental lines indicate periodic formation of cementum which can be seen best in decalcified specimen under light microscopy.

8. **A.** Enamel and cementum do not meet where enamel epithelium in the cervical portion of the root is delayed in its separation from dentin.

9. **A.** In hypophosphatasia, loosening and premature loss of anterior deciduous teeth occurs, because collagen fibers of the periodontal ligament can not be incorporated into dentin.

10. **D.** The primary function of cementum is to furnish a medium for the attachment of collagen fibers that bind the tooth to alveolar bone.

11. **A.** As the most superficial layer of cementum ages, a new layer of cementum must be deposited to keep the attachment apparatus intact. The difference in resistance of bone and cementum to pressure may be caused by the fact that bone is richly vascularized, whereas cementum is avascular.

12. **D.**   After resorption has ceased, the damage usually is repaired either by formation of acellular or cellular cementum or by alternate formation of both. Tendency to reestablish the former outline of the root surface is called anatomic repair.

13. **A.**   Incremental lines indicates periodic formation of cementum.

14. **D.**   Each Sharpley's fiber is composed of numerous collagen fibrils that pass well into the cementum.

15. **C.**   Mineralization of cementoid is a highly ordered event and not the random precipitation of ions into an organic matrix.

16. **C.**   Damage to roots such as fractures and resorptions can be repaired by the deposition of new cementum.

17. **D.**   The cells of the dental sac form the dental follicle, which forms cementoblasts.

18. **A.**   Acellular cementum usually predominates on the coronal half of the root, whereas cellular cementum is more frequent on the apical half. Cellular cementum is always thickest around the apex and, by its growth, contributes to the length of the root.

19. **C.**   Cementum is thinnest of the cementoenamel junction (20 to 50 μm) and thickest toward the apex (150 to 200 μm).

20. **B.**   Refer to answer No. 18.

21. **D.**   In approximately 60% of the teeth, cementum overlaps the cervical end of enamel for a short distance.

22. **C.**   If the cemental overgrowth occurs in nonfunctional teeth or if it is not correlated with increased function, it is termed hyperplasia.

23. **A.**   This is called as cemental hyperplasia.

 **Periodontal Ligament**

1. The periodontium comprises of how many connective tissues?
   A. 2
   B. 3
   C. 4
   D. 5

2. The functions of periodontal ligament is/are:
   A. Support and nutrition
   B. Synthesis and resorption
   C. Proprioception
   D. All of the above

3. The majority of the fibers of the periodontal ligament are:
   A. Collagen
   B. Variety of micromolecules
   C. Mesenchymal
   A. All of the above

4. The mandible consists of a series of bones united by sutures found in:
   A. Birds
   B. Orthopodes
   C. Reptiles
   D. Mammals

5. Which of the following statement(s) is/are *true*?
   A. In the reptiles the teeth are ankylosed to the bone
   B. In the mammals teeth are suspended in their socket by ligament
   C. In the reptiles growth of the mandibular body in height occurs in mandibular sutures
   D. All of the above

6. **Osteoclasts are rich in:**
   A. Alkaline phosphatase
   B. Acid phosphatase
   C. Both of the above
   D. None of the above

7. **The mast cells are characterized by numerous cytoplasmic granules. The granules have been shown to contain:**
   A. Heparin
   B. Histamine
   C. Serotonin
   D. All of the above

8. **Periodontal ligament appears to be made up of:**
   A. Type I and Type II collagen
   B. Type I and Type III collagen
   C. Type II and Type III collagen
   D. Only Type III collagen

9. **The fibers in human periodontal ligament are made up of:**
   A. Collagen
   B. Oxytalan
   C. Both of the above
   D. None of the above

10. **The fiber bundle that is most numerous and constitutes the main attachment of the tooth is:**
    A. Alveolar crest group
    B. Horizontal group
    C. Oblique group
    D. Apical group

11. **What do you know about intermediate plexus in periodontal ligament?**
    A. It may appear as fibers arising from cementum and bone joined in the midregion of the periodontal space
    B. It provides a site where rapid remodeling of fibers occurs
    C. It is an artifact arising out of the plane of section and may move from one bundle to the other
    D. All of the above

12. A particular glycoprotein which occurs in filamentous form in the periodontal ligament is called:
    A. Fibronectin
    B. Proline
    C. Hydroxyproline
    D. Chitin

13. The blood supply of periodontal ligament is derived from:
    A. Branches from apical vessels that supply dental pulp
    B. Branches from intra-alveolar vessels
    C. Branches from gingival vessels
    D. All of the above

14. Which vitamin is essential for collagen synthesis?
    A. Vitamin A
    B. Vitamin B
    C. Vitamin C
    D. Vitamin D

15. Measurements of a larger number of periodontal ligament range from:
    A. 0.01 – 0.02 mm
    B. 0.01 – 0.03 mm
    C. 0.015 – 0.038 mm
    D. 0.15 – 0.38 mm

16. The thickness of the periodontal ligament is:
    A. Less in functionless and embedded teeth
    B. More in teeth that are under excessive occlusal stresses
    C. More in functionless teeth
    D. (A) and (B) are correct

17. The periodontal ligament is synthesized from:
    A. Cementum
    B. Alveolar bone
    C. Secondary cementum
    D. Middle portion of the dental follicle

18. The cementum, periodontal ligament and alveolar bone are derived from the:
    A. Dental follicle   B. Cementoid
    C. Cementoblasts   D. Sharpey's fibers

19. **The dental follicle is a condensation of:**
    A. Mesenchymal cells surrounding the enamel organ and dental papilla
    B. Cells around the dental papilla
    C. Cells around the enamel organ
    D. Ectodermal cells surrounding the enamel organ and dental papilla

20. **The fibers forming the periodontal ligament are:**
    A. Reticular
    B. Collagen
    C. Elastin
    D. Keratin

21. **The largest group of periodontal fibers are:**
    A. The apical fibers
    B. The horizontal fibers
    C. The oblique fibers
    D. The transseptal fibers

22. **The apical group of periodontal fibers originates from the:**
    A. Cervical portion of the tooth
    B. Crest of the alveolar bone
    C. Ends of the roots
    D. Mid root region

23. **The nerves present in the periodontal ligament are:**
    A. Non-myelinated
    B. Myelinated
    C. Both (A) and (B)
    D. None

24. **The principal fibers of the periodontal ligament are attached to:**
    A. Dentin and cementum
    B. Cementum and basal bone
    C. Alveolar bone proper and cementum
    D. Supporting alveolar bone and cementum

25. **Which of the following *is NOT* a function of periodontal ligament?**
    A. Supportive   B. Nutritive
    C. Sensory   D. Defensive

26. **The periodontal ligament is thinnest in:**
    A. Apical third of the root
    B. Middle region of the root
    C. Coronal third of the root
    D. Apical foramen

27. **In a non-functioning tooth the periodontal ligament is:**
    A. Thick
    B. Thin
    C. Either of the above
    D. None of the above

28. **The periodontal ligament fibers, which hold the tooth in socket and oppose lateral forces are:**
    A. Gingival fibers
    B. Alveolar crest fibers
    C. Apical fibers
    D. Oblique fibers

ANSWERS

1. **C.** Two mineralized connective tissues are cementum and alveolar bone; and two fibrous connective tissue are periodontal ligament and the lamina propria of the gingival.

2. **D.** Synonyms of periodontal ligaments are desmodont, gomphosis, pericementum, dental periosteum, alveolodental ligament and periodontal membrane.

3. **A.** Ground substance of periodontal ligament is composed of a variety of macromolecules, the basic constituents of which are proteins and polysaccharides.

4. **C.** In the ancestral reptiles the teeth are ankylosed to the bone.

5. **D.** In the mammal, the growth of the mandibular body in height occurs by growth at the free margins of the alveolar process.

6. **B.** Acid phosphatase is contained in lysosomes.

7. **D.** Mast cell histamine plays a role in the inflammatory reaction and mast cells degranulate in response to antigen-antibody formation on their surface.

8. **B.** The fibers in human periodontal ligament are made up of collagen and oxytalan. Periodontal ligament appears to be made up predominantly of type I collagen.

9. **C.** Refer to answer No. 8.

10. **C.** Oblique fibers are attached in the cementum somewhat apically from their attachment to the bone.

11. **D.** Intermediate plexus is evidently an artifact arising out of the plane of section and may be attributable to the fact that the collagen fibers do not course only in one bundle but may move from one bundle to other.

12. **A.** Fibronectin contains chemical groups that attach to the surface of the fibroblasts and to collagen, certain proteoglycans and fibrin.

13. **D.** The arterioles and capillaries of the microcirculation ramify in the periodontal ligament, forming a rich network of arcades that is more evident in the half of the periodontal space adjacent to bone than that adjacent to cementum.

14. **C.** If an experimental animal is deprived of substances essential for collagen synthesis, such as vitamin C or protein, resorption of collagen will continue unabated, but its synthesis and replacement will be markedly reduced.

15. **D.** Periodontal ligament is thinnest in the middle region of root seems to indicate that the fulcrum of physiologic movement is in this region.

16. **D.** The thickness of the periodontal ligament seems to be maintained by the functional movements of the tooth.

17. **D.** The cells of the dental follicle differentiate into fibroblasts, which synthesized the fibers and ground substance of the periodontal ligament.

18. **A.** The cells at the dental follicle give origin to the cementoblasts, fibroblasts and osteoblasts.

19. **C.** The dental organ (enamel organ) and the Hertwig's epithelial root sheath are surrounded by condensation of cells, the dental sac. A thin layer of cells of dental sac lies adjacent to the dental organ is termed a dental follicle.

20. **B.** The fibers in human periodontal ligament are made up of collagen and oxytalan. Elastic fibers are restricted almost entirely to the walls of the blood vessels. The majority of fibers in the periodontal ligament are collagen.

21. **C.** The oblique fibers constitute the main attachment of the tooth. The transseptal ligament has a key role in maintaining tooth position.

22. **C.** Apical fibers radiate from the apical region of the root to the surrounding bone.

23. **C.** Autonomic unmyelinated small diameter fibers of periodontal ligament evidently are associated with blood

vessels. Large diameter nerve fibers appear to be concerned with discernment of touch and the small diameter ones with pain.

24. C. The principal collagen fibers are embedded into cementum on one side of the periodontal space and into alveolar bone on the outer. The embedded fibers are termed Sharpey's fibers.

25. D. The periodontal ligament has the following functions:
    1. Supportive
    2. Sensory
    3. Nutritive
    4. Homeostatic

26. B. The fulcrum of physiologic tooth movement is in the middle region of the root.

27. B. Periodontal ligament is thin in functionless and embedded teeth and wide in teeth that are under excessive occlusal stresses.

28. B. Alveolar crest fibers radiate from the crest of the alveolar process and attach themselves to the cervical part of the cementum.

1. **The main function of saliva is to:**
   A. Digest the food
   B. Kill the bacteria
   C. Clean the surfaces of teeth
   D. Lubricate the food and facilitate its swallowing

2. **Masticatory mucosa is the mucosa covering :**
   A. Gingiva   B. Alveolar mucosa
   C. Floor of mouth   D. Soft palate

3. **Which of the following is keratinized area?**
   A. Vermilion border of lip
   B. Alveolar mucosa
   C. Floor of oral cavity
   D. Inferior surface of tongue

4. **The connective tissue component of oral mucosa is termed the:**
   A. Basal layer
   B. Basement membrane
   C. Lamina propria
   D. Submucous layer

5. **A common feature of all epithelial cells is that they contain keratin. The analogous components of connective tissue cells are called:**
   A. Desmin   B. Vimentin
   C. Neural filaments   D. None of the above

6. **Lamina lucida contains:**
   A. Laminin
   B. Bullous pemphigoid antigen
   C. Antigen bound by the antibody KF-1
   D. Both (A) and (B)

7. **The percentage of cell membrane occupied by hemides-mosomes is highest in basal cells of:**
   A. Gingiva and palate
   B. Alveolar mucosa
   C. Buccal mucosa
   D. Tongue

8. **Out of the four layers which cells are the most active in protein synthesis?**
   A. Basal cells   B. Spinous cells
   C. Granular cells   D. Corneum cells

9. **Odland body is found in:**
   A. Spinous cell layers
   B. Granular cell layers
   C. Both (A) and (B)
   D. None of the above

10. **The lamina propria, a layer of dense connective tissue, is:**
    A. Thicker in anterior than in posterior parts of palate
    B. Thicker in posterior than in anterior part of palate
    C. Not found in posterior part of palate
    D. Not found in anterior part of palate

11. **Gingiva most often is:**
    A. Nonkeratinized
    B. Keratinized
    C. Orthokeratinized
    D. Parakeratinized

12. **Which of the following statement(s) is/are *correct*?**
    A. In the absence of sulcus there is no free gingiva
    B. The disappearance of stippling is an indication of gingivitis
    C. In younger females the connective tissue of gingiva is more finely textured than in the males
    D. All of the above

13. **In a three-dimensional view, the interdental papilla of posterior teeth is tent shaped, whereas in anterior teeth its shape is:**
    A. Pyramidal   B. Rectangular
    C. Elliptical   D. Square

14. The gingival 'col' is more vulnerable to periodontal disease because it is:
    A. Keratinized
    B. Parakeratinized
    C. Nonkeratinized
    D. Orthokeratinized

15. The accessory fibers that extend interproximally between adjacent teeth are known as:
    A. Transseptal fibers
    B. Dentogingival fibers
    C. Alveologingival fibers
    D. Circular fibers

16. The pigmentation is more abundant at the:
    A. Buccal gingiva
    B. Labial gingiva
    C. Base of the interdental papilla
    D. Lingual gingiva

17. The gingiva is:
    A. 75% parakeratinized
    B. 15% keratinized
    C. 10% nonkeratinized
    D. All of the above

18. The lymph supply of gingiva is:
    A. Submental
    B. Submandibular
    C. Jugulo-omohyoid
    D. Only (A) and (B)

19. Vermilion border, which is the transitional zone between the skin of the lip and the mucous membrane of the lip, is also known as:
    A. White zone
    B. Red zone
    C. Reducing zone
    D. Violet zone

20. The sebaceous glands lateral to the corner of the mouth and often seen opposite the molars are called:
    A. Fordyce's spot
    B. Hutchinson spot
    C. Intestinal polyposis
    D. Miller's spot

21. **Which papillae of tongue are keratinized and do not contain taste buds?**
    A. Fungiform papillae
    B. Filiform papillae
    C. Vallate papillae
    D. (B) and (C)

22. **Which of the following statement(s) is/are *true*?**
    A. Sweet taste is perceived at the tip of the tongue
    B. Salty taste is perceived at the lateral border of the tongue
    C. Bitter and sour taste are perceived on the palate and in the posterior part of the tongue
    D. All of the above

23. **Which statement about oral mucosa in general is not *correct*?**
    A. Oral mucosa is defined as moist lining of the oral cavity that is in continuation with the exterior surface of skin
    B. Oral mucosa is situated anatomically between the skin and intestinal mucosa. Hence, it shows some properties of both
    C. Oral mucosa shows regional structural modifications according to the stress and workload borne by it
    D. The epithelium of the oral mucosa is always ortho-keratinized

24. **The gingival sulcus is formed by the:**
    A. Tooth surface and epithelial covering of attached gingiva
    B. Tooth surface and epithelial covering of free gingiva
    C. Free gingival groove and mucogingival junction
    D. Epithelial covering of the free and attached gingiva

25. **The reduced enamel epithelium:**
    A. Is about 40 microns thick
    B. Produces the primary enamel cuticle
    C. Does not protect the enamel until tooth eruption
    D. Produces the primary attachment epithelium

26. **After tooth eruption, the reduced enamel epithelium:**
    A. Causes shrinkage of the stratum reticulum
    B. Promotes the differentiation of dentin
    C. Forms the epithelial attachment
    D. Forms the secondary enamel cuticle

27. The last organic material secreted by the ameloblast is:
    A. Primary enamel cuticle
    B. Secondary cuticle
    C. Enamel tufts
    D. Tomes' process

28. The oral epithelium is attached to the enamel via:
    A. Reticular fibers
    B. Collagen fibers
    C. Hemidesmosomes
    D. Elastic fibers

29. Oral Epithelium is:
    A. Nervous tissue
    B. Muscle tissue
    C. Connective tissue
    D. Avascular tissue

30. The lamina propria of the oral mucous membrane contains:
    A. Ectoderm
    B. Bone
    C. Keratin
    D. Blood vessels

31. Majority of taste buds are found on the:
    A. Filiform papillae
    B. Fungiform papillae
    C. Circumvallate papillae and the adjacent trench wall.
    D. All of the above

32. Glands of von Ebner empty their contents into:
    A. Fungiform papillae
    B. Circumvallate trench
    C. Filiform papilla
    D. None of the above

33. The gingival sulcus is bounded by:
    A. Free gingival groove and the junction of mucosa and gingiva
    B. Surface of the tooth and the attached gingiva
    C. Epithelial covering of the free gingiva and the tooth surface
    D. Epithelial covering of the free gingiva and the attached gingiva.

34. **The specialized mucosa is present on:**
    A. Lips and cheeks
    B. Gingiva and hard palate
    C. Dorsum of tongue and taste buds
    D. Floor of mouth and soft palate

35. **The connective tissue component of the oral mucosa is known as:**
    A. Submucosa
    B. Basal lamina
    C. Lamina propria
    D. Dermis

36. **The basement membrane of oral mucosa:**
    A. Can be seen by light microscope
    B. Is present at the interface of epithelium and connective tissue
    C. Has a width of 1-4 nm
    D. All of the above

37. **The epithelium of the oral mucous membrane is:**
    A. Stratified columnar
    B. Simple squamous epithelium
    C. Stratified squamous
    D. Non-stratified squamous

38. **The epithelium present in gingiva and hard palate is:**
    A. Parakeratinized
    B. Nonkeratinized
    C. Keratinized
    D. Any of the above

39. **The epithelium of cheek and sublingual tissue is:**
    A. Nonkeratinized
    B. Parakeratinized
    C. Keratinized
    D. None of the above

40. **Of the four layers, the cells most active in protein synthesis are of:**
    A. Stratum corneum
    B. Stratum granulosum
    C. Stratum spinosum
    D. Stratum basale

41. **The mucous membrane of the soft palate is:**
    A. Parakeratinized
    B. Nonkeratinized
    C. Keratinized
    D. Any of the above

42. **Masticatory mucosa *is NOT* present on:**
    A. Palatal fauces
    B. Attached gingiva
    C. Dorsum of the tongue
    D. Floor of the mouth

43. **Keratinosomes (Odland body) help in:**
    A. Exchange of fluids
    B. Nutrition
    C. Sensory perception
    D. Formation of intercellular agglutinating material

44. **Jacobson's organ is:**
    A. Also known as vomeronasal organ
    B. Ellipsoidal structure lined with olfactory epithelium
    C. Considered as auxiliary olfactory sense organ
    D. All the above are correct

45. **The disappearance of the stippling from the gingiva indicates:**
    A. Trauma
    B. Old age
    C. Progressive gingivitis
    D. Is a normal feature

46. **The most numerous group of gingival fibers is:**
    A. Dentoperiosteal
    B. Dentogingival
    C. Alveologingival
    D. Circular

47. **The interdental ligament is formed by:**
    A. Dentogingival fibers
    B. Dentoperiosteal fibers
    C. Transseptal fibers
    D. Alveologingival fibers

48. **A common feature of melanocytes, Langerhans cells and Merkel cell is that they all:**
    A. Produce melanin
    B. Have a low or no desmosomal attachment with surrounding keratinocytes
    C. Are dendritic
    D. Are pressure sensitive cells

49. **The Langerhans cells are:**
    A. Found in upper layers of skin and the mucosal epithelium
    B. Of hematopoietic origin
    C. Involved in the immune response
    D. All of the above

50. **Merkel cells help in:**
    A. Nutritive function
    B. Sensory function
    C. Neurosensory activities
    D. Olfactory function

51. **Number of the circumvallate papilla ranges from:**
    A. 20 to 25
    B. 15 to 20
    C. 8 to 10
    D. 4 to 5

52. **The papilla responsible to recognize sour taste is:**
    A. Vallate papilla
    B. Foliate papilla
    C. Fungiform papilla
    D. Filiform papilla

53. **Which of the followings in located at the angle of the V-shaped terminal groove?**
    A. Foramen ovale   B. Foramen cecum
    C. Foramen magnum   D. None of the above

54. **Bitter and sour taste sensations are mediated by:**
    A. Chorda tympani
    B. Hypoglossal nerve
    C. Glossopharyngeal nerve
    D. Intermediofacial nerve

ANSWERS

1. **D.** Saliva contains 25% to 30% of the total amylase protein.

2. **A.** Masticatory mucosa also covers the hard palate.

3. **A.** The epithelial tissues of the gingival and hard palate (masticatory mucosa) are keratinized.

4. **C.** The comparable part of skin is known as dermis or corium.

5. **B.** In muscle cells they are called desmin, and in nerve cells neural filaments. These all resembles tonofilaments, are 7 to 11 nm in width and can be reconstituted *in vitro* from the isolated filaments.

6. **D.** Lamina densa contains type IV collagen and an antigen bound by the antibody KF-1.

7. **A.** Hemidesmosomes anchor the cells to the basal lamina. They consist of a single attachment plaque, the adjacent plasma membrane and an associated extra-cellular structure that appears to attach the epithelium to the connective tissue.

8. **B.** Spinous cells synthesize additional proteins that differ from those made in the basal cells. This change indicates their biochemical commitment to keratinization. The basal cells and the parabasal spinous cells are referred to as the stratum germinativum.

9. **C.** They are also known as keratinosomes or membrane coating granules and contribute to the permeability barrier at the junction of granular and cornified cell layers.

10. **A.** The lamina propria may attach to the periosterum of alveolar bone, or it may overlay the submucosa.

11. **D.** In parakeratinization, the cells retain pyknotic and condensed nuclei and other partially lysed cell organells until they desquamate.

12. **D.** Stippling is functional adaptations to mechanical impacts. The disappearance of stippling is an indication

of edema, an expression of an involvement of the gingival in a progressing gingivitis.

13. **A.** When the interdental papilla is tent-shaped, the central part is like a valley; called the col. The col is more vulnerable to periodontal disease.

14. **C.** Col is a concave area and hence more plaque is deposited here.

15. **A.** These ligaments have a key role in maintaining tooth position.

16. **C.** Melanin is stored by the basal cells in the form of melanosomes, but these cells do not produce the pigment. Melanin is elaborated by melanocytes, residing in the basal layer and is transferred to the basal cells.

17. **D.** Inflammation interferes with keratinization. The more highly keratinized the tissue, the whiter and less translucent is the tissue.

18. **D.** The blood supply of gingiva is derived chiefly from the branches of the alveolar arteries.

19. **B.** The transitional region (red zone) is characterized by numerous, densely arranged long papillae of the lamina propria, reaching deep into the epithelium and carrying large capillary loops close to the surface. Thus, blood is visible through the thin parts of the translucent epithelium and gives the red color to the lips.

20. **A.** In the cheek, the mixed salivary glands are larger and are usually found between the bundles of the buccinator muscle and sometimes on its outer surface.

21. **B.** Fungiform papillae contain a few (one to three) taste buds found only on their dorsal surface.

22. **D.** Primary taste sensations are, sweet, salty, bitter and sour. Bitter taste is perceived in the middle and sour in the lateral areas of tongue.

23. **D.** The epithelium of oral mucous membrane may be keratinized, parakeratinized or nonkeratinized, depending on location.

24. B. Once the tip of the crown has emerged in the oral cavity, the reduced enamel epithelium is termed the primary attachment epithelium. At the margin of the gingiva, the attachment epithelium is continuous with the oral epithelium. As the tooth erupts, the reduced enamel epithelium grows gradually shorter and shallow groove, the gingival sulcus may develop between the gingiva and the surface of the tooth.

25. D. Once the tip of the crown has emerged, the reduced enamel epithelium is termed the primary attachment epithelium.

26. C. Refer to answer No. 25.

27. A. When the ameloblasts finish formation of the enamel matrix, they leave a thin membrane on the surface of the enamel the primary enamel cuticle. When the ameloblasts are replaced by the oral epithelium a secondary cuticle is formed.

28. C. The epithelial attachment resembles an electron microscopic basal lamina.

29. D. Epithelium has no blood vessels. It receives nutrition through diffusion from underlying connective tissues.

30. D. The connective tissue component of oral mucose is termed as the lamina propria. It may attach to the periossum of the alveolar bone, or it may overlay the submucosa.

31. C. The filiform papillae do not contain taste buds. Fungiform papillae contain a few (one to three) taste buds on the lateral surfaces of the vallate papillae; the epithelium contains numerous taste buds. Foliate papillae also contain taste buds.

32. B. von Ebner's glands serve to wash out the soluble elements of food and are the main source of salivary lipase.

33. C. The depth of the average gingival sulcus is 1.8 mm.

34. C. The covering epithelium of filiform papillae is keratinized.

35. C. At the junction of epithelium and lamina propria there is basal lamina at the electron microscopic level and the basement membrane of the light microscopic level.

36. D. Basement membrane is present within the connective tissue.

37. C. In human the epithelia of the gingival and hard palate (masticatory mucosa) are keratinized. The cheeck, facial and sublingual tissues are normally non-keratinized.

38. C. Refer to answer No. 37

39. A. Refer to answer No. 37

40. C. The protein synthesized by spinous cells differs than there made in the basal cells. This change indicates their biochemical commitment to keratinization.

41. B. When normal keratinizing tissue such as the epidermis becomes parakeratinized, it is referred to as parakeratosis.

42. C. Dorsum of tongue has specialized mucosa.

43. D. Keratinosomes (Odland body or membrane coating granules) are present in the upper spinous and granular cell layers.

44. D. Jacobson's organ (the vomeronasal organ) is a small ellipsoid (cigar shaped) structure lined with olfactory epithelium that extends from the nose to the oral cavity. In humans Jacobson's organ is apparent in the twelfth to fifteenth fetal week after which it undergoes involution.

45. C. Stippling probably is functional adaptation to masticatory impact.

46. B. Dentogingival fibers extend from the cervical cementum into the lamina propria of the gingiva.

47. C. Transseptal fibers extend interproximally between adjacent teeth.

48. B. Melanocytes are residing in the basal layer of epithelium. The Langerhans cells are found in the upper layer of skin and mucosal epithelium restricted to zones of orthokeratinization. Merkel cells are also present among basal cells.

49. D.   Langerhans cells originate in the bone marrow.

50. C.   Merkel cells are neurally interrelated, though locking neural flaments.

51. C.   Circumvallate papilla are present in front of the dividing V-shaped terminal sulues.

52. B.   Vallate papillae—for bitter taste.

Foliate papillae—for sour taste.

Fungiform papillae—for sweet taste at the tip and for salty taste at the border of tongue.

53. B.   Foramen cecum represents the remnant of the thyroglossal duct.

54. C.   Sweet and salty taste are mediated by the inter-mediofacial nerve by the chorda tympani.

Alveolus

1. **In the beginning of the second month of fetal life the skull consists of the:**
   A. Chondrocranium
   B. Desmocranium
   C. Appendicular skeleton
   D. All of the above

2. **Which bone develops in desmocranium?**
   A. Frontal bone
   B. Parietal bone
   C. Greater wing of sphenoid bone
   D. All of the above

3. **The mandible makes its appearance as a bilateral structure in the 6th week of fetal life as thin plate of bone:**
   B. Mesial to Meckel's cartilage
   C. Lateral to Meckel's cartilage
   D. Mesial and lateral to Meckel's cartilage
   E. Mesial and some distance from Meckel's cartilage

4. **Spongy bone is least found in region of:**
   A. Anterior teeth
   B. Premolar teeth
   C. Molar teeth
   D. Upper posterior teeth only

5. **The interdental and inter-radicular septa contain the perforating canals of:**
   A. Alock's
   B. Zuckerkandl and Hirschfeld
   C. Dorello's
   D. Gartner's

6. **Which enzyme participates in the deposition of hydroxy-apatite crystals in bone?**
   A. Alkaline phosphatase
   B. Adenosine triphosphatase
   C. Pyrophosphatases
   D. All of the above

7. **Osteoclasts are multinucleated giant cells formed by monocytes and are found in bay-like depression in the bone called:**
   A. Haversian canal
   B. Volkman canal
   C. Howship's lacunae
   D. Hirschfeld canal

8. **During orthodontic tooth movement on the pressure side there is an increase in the level of:**
   A. Odontoblast
   B. Cementoblast
   C. Alkaline phosphatase
   D. Cyclic adenosine monophosphophate

9. **The body of the mandible is formed by the:**
   A. Conversion of cartilage directly into bone
   B. Ordinary endochondral ossification similar to that of most long bones
   C. Intramembranous ossification similar to that of the bones of the cranial vaultv
   D. None of the above

10. **The upper jaw:**
    A. Is formed by fusion of the maxilla and premaxilla
    B. Develops from the otic capsule
    C. Is formed from Meckel's cartilage
    D. Develops from the nasolacrimal groove

11. **The mandible ossifies:**
    A. From one center in the midline of the mandible
    B. From two centers located medially to Meckel's cartilage
    C. As an endomembranous bone
    D. None of the above

12. **Which of the following is vascularized:**
    A. Cementum
    B. Enamel
    C. Bone
    D. Calculus

13. **The area of alveolar bone where Sharpey's fibers are embedded is called:**
    A. Lamellar bone
    B. Bundle bone
    C. Intramembranous bone
    D. Haversian bone

14. **Mark *the correct* statements about bundle bone. It:**
    A. Lines the socket in the teeth that are subjected to stress
    B. Anchors the Sharpey's fibers of the periodontal ligament
    C. Contains fewer matrix collagen fibrils than typical bone
    D. All of the above are correct

15. **The alveolar bone:**
    A. Consists of a compact layer and a cancellous layer
    B. Can be demarcated from the bone of the jaw
    C. Is known as periodontal plate
    D. Increases in size to compensate for loss of permanent teeth

16. **The bone consists of:**
    A. 65% organic and 35% inorganic material
    B. 65% inorganic and 35% organic
    C. 70% organic and 30% inorganic
    D. 50% organic and 50% inorganic part

17. **The cells present inside the Howships lacunae are:**
    A. Osteocytes
    B. Osteoclasts
    C. Odontoblasts
    D. Osteoblasts

ANSWERS

1. **D.** Desmocranium is membranous white, both the other are cartilogenous.

2. **D.** Intramembranous bone may develop in proximity to cartilaginous parts of the skull or directly in the membranous capsule of the brain called desmocranium.

3. **C.** The mandible develops as intramembranous bone.

4. **A.** Usually, the cortical bone is fused with the alveolar bone proper in the region of anterior teeth of both jaws.

5. **B.** These nutrient canals house the interdental and interradicular arteries, veins, lymph vessels and nerves.

6. **D.** The inorganic material of bone (65%) almost exclusively consists of calcium and inorganic orthophosphate in the form of hydroxyapatite crystals.

7. **C.** Osteoclasts are multinucleated giant cells and eliminate overage bony tissue or bone that is no longer adapted to mechanical forces. The part of it in contact with the bone shows a convoluted surface, the ruffled border, which is the site of the great activity.

8. **D.** This enzyme may play some role in bone resorption.

9. **C.** The mandible develops as intramembranous bone lateral to the cartilage of mandibular arch—Meckel's cartilage. Condyle develops by endochondral assification.

10. **A.** The human maxilla is homologus to two bones, the maxilla proper and the premaxilla. Premaxilla extends from the incisive foramen to the alveolus of the canine.

11. **B.** The mandible makes its appearance as a bilateral structure in the sixth week of fetal life as a thin plate of bone lateral to and at some distance from, Meckel's cartilage.

12. **C.** Cementum shares some physical, chemical and structural characteristics with compact bone.

13. **B.** The alveolar bone proper forms the inner wall of the and called as cribriform plate which consists partly of lamellated and partly of bundle bone. The bundle bone is characterized by the scarcity of the fibrils in the intercellular substance.

14. **D.** Since bundle bone contains more calcium salts per unit area them other types of bone tissue, such areas are seen in roentgenograms as dense radiopacities.

15. **A.** Supporting alveolar bone consists of two parts— (1) cortical plates, which consist of compact bone and form the outer and inner plates of the alveolar processes, and (2) the spongy bone, which fills the area between these plates and the alveolar bone proper.

16. **A.** The inorganic material is hydroxyapatite while the organic material is primarily type I collagen.

17. **B.** The part of the osteoclast in contact with bone shows a convoluted surface, the ruffled border, which is the site of great activity.

Salivary Glands

1. **The salivary glands are:**
   A. Exocrine
   B. Endocrine
   C. Holocrine
   D. None of the above

2. **The "basket cells" are also known as:**
   A. Myoepithelial cells
   B. Endothelial cells
   C. Parenchymal cells
   D. None of the above

3. **Myoepithelial cells are abundant in:**
   A. Sweat glands
   B. Mammary glands
   C. Both (A) and (B)
   D. None of the above

4. **Which of the following statement(s) is/are *true*?**
   A. Parotid gland is purely serous
   B. Submandibular gland is mixed but predominantly serous in nature
   C. Sublingual gland is mixed but predominantly mucous in nature
   D. All of the above

5. **The three bilaterally paired major salivary glands are located:**
   A. Extraorally
   B. Intraorally
   C. In tongue
   D. In neck

6. **The parotid glands open into the:**
   A. Stensen's duct
   B. Wharton's duct
   C. Bartholin's duct
   D. Blanden duct

7. **The parotid gland duct opens into the oral cavity at the position:**
   A. On the floor of the mouth
   B. At the side of the lingual frenum
   C. At the caruncula
   D. On the buccal mucosa opposite the maxillary 2nd molar

8. **Which statement(s) is/are *true*?**
   A. The parotid gland is purely serous
   B. In infants, few mucous secretory units may be found in parotid gland
   C. Both (A) and (B)
   D. None of the above

9. **Which gland(s) is/are pure serous in nature?**
   A. Parotid and von Ebner's glands
   B. Palatine glands only
   C. Glossopalatine glands
   D. Lingual glands

10. **Which gland(s) is/are purely mucous?**
    A. Palatine glands
    B. Glossopalatine glands
    C. Posterior lingual mucous glands
    D. All of the above

11. **The primordia of the parotid and submandibular glands appear during 6th week of fetal life, whereas the primordium of sublingual glands appears after:**
    A. 3-4th weeks of fetal life
    B. 7-8th weeks of fetal life
    C. 9-10th weeks of fetal life
    D. 10-12 weeks of fetal life

12. **The minor salivary glands begin their development in fetal life during:**
    A. 1st month B. 2nd month
    C. 3rd month D. 4th month

13. **The total volume of saliva-secreted daily is approximately:**
    A. 750 ml B. 1.5 liter
    C. 2 liter D. 3 liter

14. **The largest amount of saliva is produced by:**
    A. Submandibular gland
    B. Sublingual gland
    C. Parotid gland
    D. Lingual glands

15. **The pH of whole saliva is:**
    A. 1.2 – 2.4
    B. 3.0 – 5.6
    C. 6.7 – 7.4
    D. 7.0 – 8.2

16. **The predominant salivary immunoglobulin is:**
    A. Ig A
    B. Ig G
    C. Ig E
    D. Ig M

17. **Human parotid gland produces a hormone, which is known as:**
    A. Menotropins
    B. Parotin
    C. Serotonin
    D. Prohormone

18. **Salivary glands *are not* found in:**
    A. Anterior part of hard palate
    B. Posterior part of hard palate
    C. In mandible posterior to third molar teeth
    D. Nasopalatine canal

19. **The severance of the duct of minor salivary gland and pooling of saliva in the tissues is called as:**
    A. Ranula
    B. Mucocele
    C. Congenital epulis
    D. Sialadenitis

20. **What is the use of sialochemistry?**
    A. Determination of the quantity and composition of the saliva
    B. Determination of ovulation time
    C. Both (A) and (B)
    D. None of the above

21. **Which of the following statement(s) is/are *true* about the connective tissue elements of the salivary gland?**
    A. The connective tissue forms a distinct capsule around major glands but not around minor glands
    B. The connective tissue elements carry the vascular and nerve supply of the gland
    C. From the capsule connective tissue septa penetrate the gland subdividing it into lobules
    D. All of the above are correct

22. **'Bartholin's duct' is a secretory duct of:**
    A. Parotid gland
    B. Sublingual gland
    C. Submandibular gland
    D. Palatine glands

23. **The antibacterial proteins present in saliva is/ are:**
    A. Lysozymes
    B. Lactoferrins
    C. Both of the above
    D. None of the above

24. **The major glands may become enlarged during:**
    A. Protein deficiency
    B. Alcoholism
    C. Pregnancy
    D. All of the above

25. **Salivary flow is reduced in:**
    A. Xerostomia
    B. Sjögren's syndrome
    C. Inflammation of glands
    D. All of the above

ANSWERS

1. A. The production of the saliva is the most important function of the salivary glands.

2. A. Myoepithelial cells are closely related to the secretary and intercalated duct cells, lying between the basal lamina and the basement membranes of the parenchymal cells.

3. C. Myoepithelial cells are considered to have a contractile function, helping to expel secretions from the lamina of the secretary units and ducts.

4. D. The secretary products of most mucous cells differ from those of serous cells in two important respects:
   i. They have little or no enzymatic activity and probably serve mainly for lubrication and protection of oral tissue.
   ii. The ratio of carbohydrate to protein is greater, and larger amount of sialic acid and occasionally sulfated sugar residues are present.

5. A. Their secretions reach the mouth by variable long ducts.

6. A. It is the main excretory duct of parotid gland.

7. D. The opening is usually marked by a small papilla.

8. C. All the acinar cells are similar in structure to the serous cells.

9. A. The ducts of small serous glands called von Ebner glands are situated in to the trough of circumvallate papilla. These glands are located between the muscle fibers of the tongue below the vallate papilla. They are also called posterior lingual serous glands.

10. D. Palatine glands form glandular aggregates in the lamina propria of the postero lateral region of the hard palate and in the submucosa of the soft palate and uvula.
The anterior lingual glands (glands of Blandin and Nuhn) are located near the apex of the tongue.

11. B. During fetal life each salivary gland is formed at a specific location in the oral cavity through the growth of a bud of oral epithelium into the underlying mesenchyme.

12. **C.** Refer to answer No. 11

13. **A.** Of which about 60% is produced by the submandibular glands, 30% by the parotids, 5% or less from the sublinguals and about 7% from the minor salivary glands.

14. **A.** Refer to answer No. 13

15. **C.** pH of parotid saliva may vary from 6 to 7.8.

16. **A.** IgA is produced locally in salivary glands by plasma cells.

17. **B.** It is believed that parotin promotes the growth of mesenchymal tissues.

18. **A.** Therefore, lesions of salivary glands can occur almost anywhere within the oral cavity.

19. **B.** Obstruction of the duct of major salivary glands can be very painful and may require surgical treatment.

20. **C.** It is also useful in diagnosis of systemic and glandular diseases.

21. **D.** Both the major and minor salivary glands are composed of parenchymatus elements invested in and supported by connective tissue.

22. **B.** Bartholinis duct opens with or near the submandibular duct along the sublingual fold.

23. **C.** Lysozyme hydrolyzes the polysaccharide of bacterial cell walls resulting in cell lysis. Lactoferrin is an iron-binding protein. In the presence of specific antibody, lactoferrin that is not saturated with iron enhances the inhibitory effect of the antibody on the microorganisms.

24. **D.** The major glands, especially the parotid, may become enlarged during starvation, protein deficiency, alcoholism, pregnancy, diabetes mellitus and liver diseases.

25. **D.** Reduction in salivary flow is most often seen in patients with sicca syndrome or Sjögren syndrome, after irradiation of the head and neck region or because of use of various therapeutic pharmacologic agents.

29 Eruption of Teeth and Physiologic Tooth Movements

1. The permanent incisors and canine first develop:
   A. Labial to deciduous tooth germs
   B. Lingual to the deciduous tooth germs
   C. Mesial to deciduous tooth germs
   D. Distal to deciduous tooth germs

2. The upper permanent molars develop in tuberosity of the maxilla and in the beginning their occlusal surface faces:
   A. Labially
   B. Lingually
   C. Mesially
   D. Distally

3. At first, the occlusal surface of the permanent mandibular molars faces:
   A. Mesially
   B. Distally
   C. Lingually
   D. Labially

4. Successional teeth possess an additional anatomic feature, the gubernacular canal and its contents, the gubernacular cord. The function of gubernacular cord is:
   A. Guiding the permanent tooth as it erupts
   B. Blood supply to tooth
   C. Blood supply to bone
   D. Nutrition to tooth

5. Removal of the root:
   A. Prevents eruption of tooth
   B. Does not prevent eruption
   C. Causes regeneration of root
   D. None of the above

6. **Which ligament has a key role in maintaining tooth position?**
   A. Horizontal group ligament
   B. Apical group ligament
   C. Inter-radicular group ligament
   D. Transseptal ligament

7. **Clinically as the teeth break through the oral mucosa, there is often some pain, slight fever, and general malaise, all signs of an inflammatory process. In infants, these symptoms are popularly called:**
   A. Teething   B. Biting
   C. Erythroblastosis fetalis   D. Erythema multiforme

8. **Resorption of the roots of the deciduous incisors and canines begins on their:**
   A. Mesial surface   B. Distal surface
   C. Labial surface   D. Lingual surface

9. **The most likely cause of tooth eruption is:**
   A. The growing root
   B. Vascular pressure
   C. The developing periodontal ligament
   D. Bone growth

10. **The transseptal ligament connects:**
    A. Cementum to bone
    B. Bone to bone
    C. Gingiva to cementum
    D. Cementum of one tooth to the cementum of adjacant tooth

11. **The actual eruptive movements occur mainly:**
    A. In a horizontal direction
    B. In a rotational direction
    C. In an axial direction
    D. In multiple directions

12. **Which one of the following events does not take place during the active phase of eruption?**
    A. Bone deposition and resorption on the crypt wall
    B. Root formation
    C. Organization of a periodontal ligament from the dental follicle
    D. Gradual separation of the attachment epithelium from the enamel surface

13. **Prior to actual eruption in the jaw bone, the tooth:**
    A. Rotates
    B. Moves in an apical direction
    C. Moves in a horizontal direction
    D. Moves in multiple directions

14. **In the teeth with deciduous predecessors which canal is present that has an influence on eruptive tooth movement:**
    A. Accessory canal
    B. Gubernacular canal
    C. Incisive canal
    D. Nasolacrimal canal

ANSWERS

1. **B.** Because they develop from a lingual extension of the free end of the dental lamina opposite to the enamel organ of each deciduous teeth.

2. **D.** The permanent teeth without deciduous predecessors also move from the site of their initial differentiation. These movements are linked to jaw growth.

3. **A.** Refer to answer No. 2.

4. **A.** They may have an influence on eruptive tooth movement.

5. **B.** Onset of eruptive tooth movement is probably coincident with periodontal ligament formation. If root formation is responsible for eruption and then the onset of root formation and eruptive movement would coincide. Indeed, initial root formation results in bone resorption at the base of the socket. Some teeth move a greater distance than the length of their fully formed roots and others still erupt after root formation have been completed.

6. **D.** Transseptal ligaments run between teeth across the alveolar process. The mesial drift is achieved by occlusal forces.

7. **A.** When a tooth breaks through the oral epithelium an acute inflammatory response occurs in the connective tissue adjacent to the tooth, even in the germ-free animals.

8. **D.** Refer to answer No. 7

9. **C.** Eruptive movement is brought about by a combination of events involving a force initiated by fibroblasts of the periodontal ligaments.

10. **D.** The mesial drift is achieved by contraction of transseptal fibers and enhanced by occlusal forces.

11. **C.** However, it is important that jaw growth is normally occurring while most teeth are erupting, so that movement in planes other than axial (occlusal) is superimposed on eruptive movement.

12. **D.** In passive eruption, gradual separation of the attachment epithelium from the enamel surface takes place.

13. **D.** The growth in the length of the infant jaws provides room for the tooth germ to drift. At the same fome this tooth germ also move as the jaws increase in width and height.

14. **B.** Gubernacular canal contains gubernacular cord, which may have a function in guiding the permanent tooth as it erupts.

 **Shedding of
Deciduous Teeth**

1. Resorption of the roots of the deciduous incisors and canines begins on their:
   A. Mesial surface
   B. Distal surface
   C. Labial surface
   D. Lingual surface

2. Resorption of the roots of deciduous molars often first begins on their:
   A. Outer surface
   B. Inner surface
   C. Mesial surface
   D. Distal surface

3. A characteristic feature of the odontoclast is high level of activity of the enzyme which is known as:
   A. Alkaline phosphatase
   B. Acid phosphatase
   C. Pyrophosphatase
   D. Hyaluronidase

4. When a successional tooth germ is missing, shedding of deciduous tooth is:
   A. Premature
   B. Normal
   C. Delayed
   D. Never

5. Sometimes part of the roots of deciduous teeth are not in the path of erupting permanent teeth and may escape resorption. They are most frequently found in association with the permanent:
   A. Incisors   B. Canine
   C. Premolars   D. Molars

6. **Retained deciduous teeth are most often the upper:**
   A. Central incisor
   B. Lateral incisor
   C. Canine
   D. Molar

7. **For the removal of the dental hard tissues the cells responsible are:**
   A. Odontoclast
   B. Osteoclasts
   C. Osteocytes
   D. Chondroblast

8. **A high level of enzyme acid phosphatase is a characteristic feature of:**
   A. Mast cells
   B. Osteoclast
   C. Osteocytes
   D. Chondrocyte

9. **The result of premature loss of deciduous teeth is:**
   A. Delayed eruption of successor
   B. Earlier eruption of successor
   C. No effect on eruption
   D. Eruption does not occur

ANSWERS

1. **D.** The pressure generated by the growing and erupting permanent tooth dictates the pattern of deciduous tooth resorption. This pressure is directed against the lingual root surfaces of the decidous anterior teeth.

2. **B.** The early developing premolars are found between the roots of deciduous molars.

3. **B.** Odontoclasts are responsible for the removal of dental hard tissues and are identical to osteoclasts.

4. **C.** It seems clear that pressure from the erupting suceessional tooth plays a key role because the odontoclasts differentiate at predicated sites of pressure. Although pressure obviously has a key role in initiating tooth resorption , other factors may also be involved, because removal of the permanent tooth germ delays, but does not prevent shedding of its deciduous predecessor.

5. **C.** Such remnants, consisting of dentine and cementum, may remain embedded in the jaw for a considerable time. They are most frequently found in the region of lower second premolars because the roots of the lower second deciduous molar are strongly curved or divergent.

6. **B.** Such teeth are usually permanent successors or their successors are impacted. Order of retain teeth is as follows:

   Upper lateral incisor > second permanent premolar (Mandibular > lower central incisor)

7. **A.** Odontoclasts are identical to osteoclasts, the cells responsible for the removal of bone.

8. **B.** This is also a characterstic feature of odontoclasts.

9. **C.** Premature loss of deciduous tooth may lead to early eruption of its successor. Situations such as loss of deciduous tooth and drifting of adjacent tooth cause delayed eruption of permanent tooth.

31 Temporomandibular Joint

1. **The condylar cartilage is:**
   A. Both primary and secondary cartilages
   B. A primary cartilage present prior to ossification of the mandible
   C. A secondary cartilage not present prior to ossification of the mandible
   D. A secondary cartilage present prior to ossification of the mandible

ANSWER

1. **C.** Condyle develops by endochondral growth that is by growth of the hyaline cartitage.

 Maxillary Sinus

1. The maxillary sinus communicates with the environment by:
   A. Superior nasal meatus
   B. Middle nasal meatus
   C. Middle nasal meatus and the nasal vestibule
   D. Inferior nasal meatus

2. Maxillary sinus epithelium is:
   A. Stratified and columnar
   B. pseudostratified columnar and ciliated
   C. Squamous and nonciliated
   D. Glandular

3. The secretory cells present in the sub-epithelial glands of maxillary sinus are:
   A. Mucous cells
   B. Serous cells
   C. Both of the above
   D. None of the above

4. All are the functions of the maxillary sinus *except:*
   A. Protect the internal structures against exposure to cold air
   B. Contribute resonance to voice
   C. Production of bactericidal lysozyme
   D. Helps in mastication

ANSWERS

1. **C.**   The maxillary sinus is established in the embryo of about 32 mm CRL (crown-rump-length).

2. **B.**   Maxillary sinus epithelium is derived from the olfactory epithelium of the middle nasal meatus.

3. **C.**   Mucous producing cells are secretory goblet cells.

4. **D.**   Sinuses also reduce the weight of the skull.

33 Advanced Techniques in the Study of Oral Tissues

1. **Which statement(s) is/are *true*?**
   - A. Hyaluronic acid predominates in the loose connective tissues
   - B. Hyaluronic acid has high capacity to bind water and is responsible for transport and diffusion of metabolic substances across tissue
   - C. Bacterial infections may occur as a result of the hydrolytic action of the bacterial enzyme hyaluronidase
   - D. All of the above

2. **The organic components of bone are mainly:**
   - A. 93% type I collagen
   - B. Hydroxyapatite
   - C. 90% type II collagen
   - D. 90% type IV collagen

3. **Which is considered to be one of the most ideal fixatives?**
   - A. Sodium hypochlorite
   - B. Formaldehyde
   - C. Acetyldehyde
   - D. H_2SO_4

4. **Formaldehyde as a fixative is generally used as a:**
   - A. 10 % solution
   - B. 20 % solution
   - C. 30 % solution
   - D. 40 % solution

5. **Rossman's fluid contains:**
   - A. Formaldehyde
   - B. Alcohol
   - C. Picric acid and acetic acid
   - D. All of the above

6. **Carnoy's mixture, is composed of:**
   A. Ethyl alcohol
   B. Acetic acid
   C. Chloroform
   D. All of the above

7. **Feulgen's reaction is used for visualizing:**
   A. DNA
   B. RNA
   C. Chromosome
   D. Microsome

8. **The best known and frequently used technique for detection of carbohydrate grouping is:**
   A. Versene technique
   B. PAS technique
   C. Carnoy's mixture
   D. All of the above

9. **Which is nonreactive with PAS method?**
   A. Developing bone
   B. Resorbing bone
   C. Resorbing dentin
   D. Enamel matrix

10. **Which type of collagen is absent in normal adult dentin?**
    A. Type I
    B. Type II
    C. Type III
    D. All of the above

11. **The localization of type III collagen in dentin is found in:**
    A. Dentinogenesis imperfecta type II
    B. Osteogenesis imperfecta
    C. None of the above
    D. Both (A) and (B)

12. **In the developing molar and incisor teeth, alkaline phosphatase is present in the:**
    A. Outer enamel epithelium
    B. Inner enamel epithelium
    C. Stellate reticulum
    D. Stratum intermedium

13. **The lack of mast cells is found in:**
    A. Tongue
    B. Gingiva
    C. ANUG
    D. All of the above

14. **Elevation of which enzyme is considered to assist in the diagnosis of cancer?**
    A. Amylase
    B. Glucose-6-phosphate dehydrogenase
    C. Aminopeptidase
    D. Cytochrome oxidase

ANSWERS

1. **D.** Hyaluronic acid is synthesized as a very large, free nonsulfated GAG (glycosaminoglycan) that does not require a protein core and differs from chondroitin sulfates in having acetylglucosamines instead of acetylgalactosamines as its constituents.

2. **A.** Bone consists of about 65% inorganic and 35% organic material. The inorganic material is hydroxyapatits while the organic material is primarily type I collagen, which lies in a ground substance of glycoproteins and proteoglcans.

3. **B.** This is because of its ability to react with major reactive groups of proteins to form polymeric or macromolecular networks, without affecting their native reactivity to histochemical procedures.

4. **A.** Formaldehyde is generally used as a 10% solution buffered to pH 7 at cold temperature in the range of 0 to 4 degree C.

5. **D.** Rossman's fluid is used for visualization of glycogen, glycoproteins and proteoglycans.

6. **D.** Carnoy's mixture is used for histochemical staining of nucleic acid.

7. **A.** Feulgen's reaction requires acid hydrolysis of the DNA polymers to expose the deoxyribose sugar residues of DNA molecules.

8. **B.** The chemical basis of this method lies in the fact that periodic acid oxidizes the glycol groups to aldehydes.

9. **D.** The PAS method is employed more than any other in studying the ground substance of teeth and bones. Under specific conditions, this method is believed to demonstrate the carbohydrate moiety as well as the glycoprotein complexes. Enamel matrix is essentially nonreactive with the PAS method. However, enamel lamellae are intensely stained in ground sections.

10. **C.** The presence of a bluish brown opalescence and a diminished pulpal chamber in the teeth of patients with dentinogenesis imperfecta type II or in osteogenesis imperfecta is associated with the realization of type III collagen in dentin.

11. **D.** Refer to answer No. 10

12. **D.** Also present in the odontoblasts, Korff's fibers and the ground substance. Alkaline phosphatase is observed to be associated with osteogenesis and dentinogenesis.

13. **C.** Mast cells are characterized by numerous cytoplasmic granules containing heparin, histamine and in some animals serotonin.

14. **B.** The levels of this enzyme become highly elevated in malignant dysplastic lesions of the oral mucosa.

Miscellaneous

1. **In which part of oral cavity mucous membrane is the thinnest?**
   A. Soft palate
   B. Labial mucosa
   C. Floor of mouth
   D. Buccal mucosa

2. **The average diameter of coronal dentinal tubules near the pulp is:**
   A. 0.2-0.5 microns
   B. 2-3 microns
   C. 0.2-0.3 microns
   D. 4-7 microns

3. **What is the thickness of the layer of prismless enamel found in primary teeth?**
   A. 25 microns
   B. 50 microns
   C. 75 microns
   D. 100 microns

4. **Desmodont is another name for:**
   A. The tooth with one wall pocket
   B. Tooth with three walled pocket
   C. Periodontal ligament
   D. Dehiscence

5. **Relative to primary mandibular incisors, permanent mandibular incisors erupt:**
   A. Lingually
   B. Facially
   C. Distally
   D. Mesially

6. **Which is the predominant factor in the formation of the alveolar process?**
   A. Eruption of teeth
   B. Normal process of growth
   C. Lengthening of the condyle
   D. Overall growth of the bodies of the maxilla and the mandible

ANSWERS

1. **C.** Histologically mucosa of the floor of mouth is non-keratinized, thinnest and loosely adherent to the underlying structures. Loose attachment to the underlying tissue provide free mobility to the tongue.

2. **B.** The dentinal tubules are approximately one micron in diameter at their outer end and 1.5 to 3.0 micron near pulpal end.

3. **A.** A relatively structure less layer of enamel, approximately 30 μm thick has been described in 70% of permanent teeth and all deciduous teeth. This structureless enamel is found least often over the cusp tips and most commonly toward the cervical areas of the enamel surface. It is also somewhat more mineralized than the bulk of the enamel beneath it. In this surface layer no prism outlines are visible.

4. **C.** Desmodont, gomphosis and periodontal membrane are synonyms of periodontal ligament.

5. **A.** Before the permanent incisors erupt the deciduous incisor must be exfoliated. This takes place by the resorption of deciduous roots. Pressure is exerted by the permanent tooth bud, which are placed lingually. The permanent mandibular incisors erupt lingually while permanent maxillary incisors erupt facially, to their respective deciduous tooth.

6. **A.** It is the tooth eruption, which play predominant role in the formation of alveolar process.